Essentials of Ferrets
A Guide for Practitioners

An Update to
A Practitioner's Guide to
Rabbits and Ferrets

Karen Purcell, DVM
Abbott Valley Veterinary Center
Cumberland, Rhode Island

Susan A. Brown, DVM, author 1st edition
Midwest Bird & Exotic Animal Hospital
Westchester, Illinois

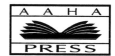
AAHA PRESS

Essentials of Ferrets
A Guide for Practitioners

An Update to *A Practitioner's Guide to Rabbits and Ferrets*

Many thanks to the AAHA Press Editorial Advisory Board:
Dr. Laurel Collins, ABVP
Dr. Richard Goebel
Dr. Charles Hickey
Dr. Clayton McKinnon
Dr. Richard Nelson, ABVP
Dr. Hal Taylor

AAHA Press
12575 W. Bayaud Avenue
Lakewood, Colorado 80228

Cover Illustration by Julie Porter

ISBN 0-941451-73-9

With thanks to my husband Denis and my parents, for all their support. And to Kathy, for making me believe that phone message!

Contents

Foreword,
2nd Edition

In 1992, when I did the research for and wrote the ferret section of the first AAHA edition of *A Practitioner's Guide to Rabbits and Ferrets* (published in 1993), there were still large gaps in the published information available on the wide range of diseases I was seeing in pet ferrets in practice. In the five years since that first AAHA book was published, there has been an explosion of published papers on this species. The majority of this material still leans heavily toward anecdotal clinical experiences; however, increased interest in the veterinary community is finally resulting in a number of sound, scientifically based research projects on the pet ferret. It is hoped that this trend toward scientifically organized scrutiny will continue to gain momentum so that the veterinary community can increase its understanding of the ferret and thus be able to manage this species' diseases more effectively.

When it came time to write this second edition, sadly my life did not allow the time needed to fulfill this commitment. Because AAHA had designed this series to be readable and applicable to the practitioner, the search went out to find someone who could do the job. So many of my "seasoned" colleagues in the exotic animal field were already overwhelmed with time commitments because there are still a small number of us performing an ever-expanding volume of work in practice, lecturing, writing, and research. Karen Purcell is a relative newcomer to this field but has demonstrated a sincere and enthusiastic commitment to her ferret patients and to the writing of this second edition. Karen has done an excellent job pulling together data from all sources, combining established concepts with new ideas, and condensing it down to a practical text for the practitioner. I had the opportunity to review her work and together we fine-tuned the material to produce a book that is worthy to take its place among other important published works on the ferret.

This book will be useful to both the veterinarian and the veterinary student in studying all aspects of the pet ferret from husbandry to the medical and surgical treatment of disease. For those wishing to obtain more information on a particular topic, there is an extensive list of references at the end of the book plus a new section, Resources, that lists a variety of valuable publications. All sections of the book have been reorganized, expanded, and updated from the first edition and contain a wealth of new information. Becoming familiar with the material in this book is an important step toward becoming an experienced practitioner with ferrets.

In conclusion, I would like to state my philosophy concerning what makes a truly exceptional veterinary practitioner in the field of ferret (and indeed all of exotic animal) medicine. There are two basic characteristics. The first characteristic is a sincere interest in and compassion for the ferret. Even if a practitioner is highly technically skilled, without a sincere interest in the species at hand it is likely that many of the subtle signs of disease will be missed, which can adversely affect the success of therapy. Economic gain should never be the primary motivation for treating these special creatures. Second, good critical thinking skills, the basis of all good medicine, should be incorporated daily in practice. Education is essential and is never ending through published material such as this book, seminars, and networking with other knowledgeable veterinarians. All of this information is critically valuable; however, we must remember that the majority of it still remains primarily anecdotal and therefore could change in a day, a month, or a year. There are no true "experts" in this field because too much is still unknown. Critical thinking allows the blending of all sources of information in order to make the best possible clinical choices.

Oh, and one more thing: you need a good sense of humor to treat ferrets. You can learn the healing and rejuvenating effects of laughter if you let the ferret's playful and often mischievous spirit into your heart. I hope that this book will reveal even this aspect of the ferret's nature to you and help you not only become more proficient in treating ferrets but also enjoy yourself along the way.

Susan A. Brown, DVM

General Information

The Veterinarian and Ferrets

Ferrets have become popular companion animals in the United States, and they are increasing in popularity throughout the world. There is a growing need for veterinarians to offer their medical and surgical skills to this booming population. Ferret owners are often as emotionally attached to their pets as are other companion animal clients and demand the same level of quality care and attention. Many of the same skills learned for dogs and cats can be applied to ferrets once their diverse medical needs are understood. Adding ferrets to any small animal practice brings both challenges and rewards to each day.

In the United States there are varying laws regarding the legality of owning ferrets. At the time of this writing, ferrets are listed as wild animals in most state conservation and wildlife codes.[1] State permits may be required to keep ferrets legally as pets or to breed them. Quarantine laws regarding bite incidents differ as well. In some states and cities it is illegal to own a ferret, and veterinary licensure may be revoked if a ferret is treated under any circumstances. These laws have been rapidly changing over the past 10 years as grassroots efforts to legalize ferrets have achieved success. Although it is impossible to explore the legal ramifications of ferret practice in these pages, it is important to be familiar with the laws in your area.

Sources of Information

Ferret owners range from the uninformed to those who own every book available on the subject. The need for information on ferret care has grown faster than veterinarians have been able to find answers. It is important to consult the information increasingly available in various media to stay informed. A number of books have been published

---

SPECIALIZED EQUIPMENT

GENERAL HOSPITAL SUPPLIES

Bitter Apple (Grannick, Cos Cob, CT) or Bitter Orange (Arc Laboratories, Atlanta, GA)

Prescription a/d Diet (Hill's Pet Products, Topeka, KS)

Deliver 2.0 (Mead Johnson Nutritionals, Evansville, IN)

Sustacal or Ensure (Abbott Laboratories, Columbus, OH)

Liver-flavored syrup for compounding medications

Fatty acid supplements

Feline hairball remedy

Small feline nail clippers

Catheter-tipped feeding syringes (20 cc)

Tabletop gram scale*

Incubator

Towels

Water bottles

Food blender

CLINICAL TECHNIQUE SUPPLIES

Small-gauge needles (20–27 gauge)

Small intravenous (IV) catheters (23–25 gauge, ¾ in.)

Spinal needles (20–22 gauge, 1½ in.) for intraosseous (IO) catheters

Syringe pump for administering measured amounts of fluids

Insulin (0.5 cc), tuberculin (TB) (1.0 cc), and 3-cc syringes

Specialized urinary catheters (Cook Veterinary Products Inc., Bloomington, IN)

Small blood containers

IV line clamps

continued

ANESTHESIA SUPPLIES

2.0–3.5 noncuffed endotracheal tubes
or silicon-cuffed tubes

Small short-bladed laryngoscope

Anesthetic face masks (custom
or small dog)

Isoflurane vaporizer with
nonrebreathing assembly

SURGICAL SUPPLIES

Hemostatic clips, small and medium

Water-circulating heating pad

Anesthetic monitoring devices (e.g.,
Doppler, pulse oximeter, respiratory
monitor)

Surgical magnification (e.g., head
loupe) (MDS, Inc., Brandon, FL, or
SurgiTelR-General Scientific Corp.,
Ann Arbor, MI)

Small surgical instruments (e.g.,
ophthalmic, microsurgery), including
Alm retractors, Heiss blunt retractors

Neonatal Satinsky vena cava clamp

Nexaband (CRx Medical, Raleigh, NC)
or Vetbond (Animal Care Products/
3M, St. Paul, MN)

Gelfoam (The Upjohn Co.,
Kalamazoo, MI)

Surgicel (Johnson & Johnson Healthcare Systems, Piscataway, NJ)

Small synthetic absorbable suture
materials (4–0 to 10–0)

Note: Manufacturers are listed only
when known to be the only source
for the equipment listed.

*Because ferrets weigh between 0.5
and 2 kg, a small gram scale with
a sturdy basket should be used for
accurate weighing. Ferrets may show
illness only by slight decreases in
weight, so accuracy is important.

in the past few years that expand on our knowledge of ferrets. Many professional journals now regularly carry articles on ferrets, as well. The Internet has a variety of sources of information, especially through consultation with other ferret-knowledgeable veterinarians. Although anecdotal evidence must be weighed carefully and misinformation is rampant, having access to the experiences of other professionals as well as owners provides a good base of information on the problems inherent in the species. See Resources for a list of information sources on ferrets. In addition, there is an increasing emphasis on small mammal medicine at veterinary conferences.

For legal information, consult your local veterinary medical association or fish and wildlife department. Be aware that the public health department of your state may have a separate set of regulations regarding ferrets, which can be confusing.

Equipment Needed

Generally, the equipment already present in most small animal practices can be used with ferrets. See chart of specialized equipment on pages 1 and 2 for helpful instrumentation.

2

Biology and Husbandry

Natural History

Mustela putorius furo, commonly known as the domestic ferret, has been part of human life for approximately 2000 years.[1] Ferrets are a member of the family Mustelidae, order Carnivora.[2] They are descended from either the European polecat (*Mustela putorius*) or the steppe polecat (*Mustela eversmanni*).[1] Other relatives include the North American black-footed ferret, otters, ermine, mink, and martens.[2] Originally domesticated for rodent control, ferrets are still used in rodent and rabbit hunting in England, Europe, and Australia, and they are raised for fur.[1]

The domestic ferret is bred to produce several color and coat variations. The natural or wild coloring of the ferret is sable, known as "fitch" in Europe, which includes dark brown or black guard hair on the extremities, a dark brown or black mask on the face, lighter brown guard hair on the trunk, and a cream-colored undercoat (figure 1). The albino ferret, which also occurs naturally, has a white coat and lack of pigment in the iris (figure 2). In the United States, more than 20 other recognized colors of ferrets have been created. These include various shades of silver (the brown guard hairs are absent, with only the cream undercoat and gray and black guard hairs remaining) (figure 3), pandas (the head and neck are white, and the body may be any shade), black or dark-eyed whites (the body hair is white, as in albinos, but the irises are pigmented), and cinnamon (a beige overall coat color) (figure 4), to name a few. Body types include "bulldog," with a flattened, thick head and body, and "whippet," with a narrow, pointed head and thin body. European breeders have produced angora ferrets, which are larger than the North American stock and have thick, long coats.

3

Behavior as Pets

Ferrets are lively and comical in their movements. They expend a
great deal of energy when they are playing and then sleep soundly for
long periods (14–16 hours daily is common). They are extremely
inquisitive and intelligent, finding ways to open cabinets and climb to
great heights. It is very important that any enclosure designed for ferrets have secure doors and openings less than 2.2 cm square to avoid
escapes.

Ferrets are easily stimulated, displaying hair elevation, leaping in the
air, and vocalizing with a "dooking" or "chattering" sound when
excited or startled. This activity can lead to traumatic injury, because
they can fall from an elevated surface. A ferret in this state may lunge
as part of its play behavior; however, this is rarely meant as aggression. Play in young ferrets also involves nipping. Nipping seldom
breaks the skin, but occasionally a ferret will bite with force. Applying
pressure on the philtrum or at the temporal-mandibular junction or
placing a drop of isopropyl alcohol in the mouth will cause release
without harm to the ferret. When ferrets exhibit fear behavior, they
back into a corner, hiss, or scream. Fearful ferrets twist and struggle
vigorously when held. If there is any danger of the ferret falling or
escaping, capture it in a soft towel and place it in a cage for a few
minutes to allow it to calm down.

New owners are frequently concerned about the odor of the ferret. The
body odor is under the control of androgynous hormones, which affect
the sebaceous secretions of the skin, and is most noticeable in the
sexually active intact male ferret. The female ferret in estrus also produces a strong body odor. The anal glands contribute little to this odor.
Ferrets do not spray anal gland contents as skunks do, and once they
have reached adulthood they do not release the anal gland material
routinely. Therefore, removing the anal glands is an unnecessary procedure in ferrets and in fact does nothing to remove overall body odor.
Neutered ferrets still retain a "musky" body odor. As with any pet,
owners should be willing to accept the animal with its peculiarities,

such as odor and behavior. Bedding should be washed twice weekly to control odor in the environment. Ferrets do not need routine bathing; however, owners who wish to bathe their pets should do so no more than once every 4 to 6 weeks with a mild pet shampoo. Flea shampoos are not recommended because they dry the haircoat excessively and may cause chemical toxicities in the animal.

Physical Characteristics

Ferrets have elongated tubular bodies with a long neck and trunk and short legs. The body size of intact males (hobs) is normally twice that of intact females (jills). Males can range in weight from 1 to 2 kg and females from 0.5 to 1.0 kg. Ferrets reach their adult size by 6 months of age.[3] Female ferrets that are neutered before weaning (sprites) tend to be larger than the average intact female. Males neutered in this manner (gibs) tend to be smaller than the average intact male. In addition, all male ferrets neutered prior to sexual maturity fail to develop the heavy neck and shoulder muscling typical of the intact male ferret.[4]

There is a normal 20 to 40% weight fluctuation during the year, especially in intact animals, due to changes in the amount of subcutaneous fat present.[5] Weight is gained in the fall and then lost in the spring. Hair molt also happens at these times. The shedding is gradual, but occasionally it can be quite dramatic with the entire undercoat coming to the surface over a 24-hour period. When a ferret has been shaved, as in the case of surgery, the hair may regrow very slowly (complete regrowth can take up to 3 months). In addition, the skin may develop a dark blue appearance just before the hair returns. The dark blue is caused by the presence of hair emerging from the follicles. Ferret markings, including mask configuration and overall hair length, shade, or texture, may change with each shed, and this is normal.[6] If there are areas of alopecia, if the coat is dry and brittle, or if the ferret is experiencing pruritus, the possibility of disease (particularly endocrine) should be investigated.

BIODATA: FERRETS[5,8,9]	
Body wt., male	1.0–2.5 kg
Body wt., female	0.5–1.5 kg
Birth weight	6–12 g
Life span (U.S.)	5–11 yrs (avg.)
Food consumption	40–70 g/day
Breeding onset, female	4.5–10 mos
Breeding onset, male	9 mos
Cycle length	induced ovulators
Gestation	42 ±2 days
Litter size	1–17 (8 average)
Weaning age	6–8 wks
Rectal temperature	100–103°F (37.8–40°C)
Respiratory rate	33–36 breaths/min
Heart rate	200–400 beats/min

Ferrets have some unique anatomical features. As the discussion here is not all-inclusive, further study is recommended before treating this species. Ferrets have very flexible spines that allow them to turn their bodies 180°. They have 7 cervical, 15 thoracic, 5 to 7 lumbar, 3 sacral, and 18 caudal vertebrae.[7] Ferrets are obligate carnivores with a simple stomach; they have no appendix or cecum. There is poor differentiation of the small and large intestines histopathologically.[7] The heart is located between the sixth and eighth ribs.[7] Male ferrets have a J-shaped os penis and prostate tissue at the base of the bladder surrounding the urethra.[7] The female has a bicornate uterus with long horns and a short body.[7]

Handling

Gentle restraint is usually all that is needed to handle a ferret. Young ferrets may be more fractious and may require firmer handling, but the average adult ferret in the United States is a docile creature.[10] It is not necessary to use gloves. A small bottle of a bitter-tasting nontoxic substance, such as Bitter Apple (Grannick, Cos Cob, CT) or isopropyl alcohol, should be kept nearby. A drop applied to the gums will induce the pet to release a bite. Pressure on the philtrum or at the temporal-mandibular junction will also cause release without harm to the ferret. To minimize bite incidents, spray the bitter-tasting substance on your hands before handling a fractious or "nipping" patient. Do not put unfamiliar ferrets up to your face, because ferrets have poor eyesight and may view the human nose as an exciting new toy!

A common method of restraining a ferret is called "scruffing" and it has a calming effect on most ferrets.[11] The technique is simple. Grasp as much skin as possible over the back of the ferret's neck (starting between the ears) and allow the lower feet to hang suspended over the examination table (figure 5). Gently stroke the abdomen to aid in relaxing the pet. Always warn the client before picking up a pet in this manner, because it may appear uncomfortable. In this position, the ferret's ears can be cleaned, nails clipped, head and ears examined, abdomen palpated, and thorax auscultated. Treats such as a feline hair-ball laxative or liquid fatty acid supplements are useful as a distraction during unpleasant procedures such as nail clipping.[11] Avoid sugar-based treats if an accurate blood glucose level is needed. Ferrets often continuously yawn when being scruffed, allowing visualization of the mouth.

Another method of restraint for examination involves tucking the ferret's body under your arm and along your side with the back of the ferret's head held in the palm of your hand (figure 6). This is a good position in which to give oral medications and to examine the head and mouth. Hold the ferret with one hand around the neck and the other firmly in front of the hind legs around the lower abdomen to give injections to a fractious animal. This can also be done with a cross-handed grip. An assistant uses the right hand to encircle the neck of the ferret with the thumb and forefinger. The left hand crosses over the body and encircles the ferret anterior to the pelvis with the thumb and forefinger. This provides a firm hold while the doctor is examining or treating an active patient.[10] A final method of restraint of the fractious ferret involves grasping the thorax from the front with your palm facing the ferret and your index finger and thumb encircling one front leg while your fourth and fifth fingers encircle the other front leg. In this way the ferret cannot turn or lower its head to bite your hand.[12]

Housing

House ferrets indoors or outdoors in areas that do not experience extremes in temperature. Rabbit- or cat-sized cages approximately 24 x 24 x 18 inches high are the *minimum* size suitable for up to two ferrets. The sides may be wire, with holes no larger than 1.0 x 0.5 inches. The floor may be either 0.25-inch wire mesh or solid metal. If the cage is outdoors, provide a sheltered area with solid walls and floor. Do not use wood for flooring because it is difficult to clean and retains odors. Pine and cedar shavings should be avoided, as dust and aromatic oils may cause respiratory irritation. Solid plastic flooring such as that found in pet carriers can lead to foot irritation; however, linoleum or no-wax flooring is acceptable. Ferrets can become hyperthermic at temperatures above 80°F (27°C), especially with high humidity, so the cage should be placed in a cool area during the summer months.[13]

Female and small male ferrets may be able to squeeze through the bars of the average metal-barred dog or cat cage in the hospital. Placing a piece of Plexiglas over the bars attached with Velcro strips or wiring wire mesh to the cage front makes an adequate modification to prevent escapes. A low litter box can be provided for elimination, although most ferrets choose a corner and use the cage papers. A water bottle or heavy bowl should be provided, preferably with water from the ferret's home. Ask the owners to provide food so that dietary changes are minimized. Attach food and water containers to the cage to prevent tipping, or use heavy crock bowls. Keep Prescription Diet a/d (Hill's Pet Products, Topeka, KS), poultry-based baby foods, Deliver 2.0 (Mead-Johnson Nutritionals, Evansville, IN), and Sustacal or Ensure (Abbott Laboratories, Columbus, OH) available in the hospital for patients that are unable to eat solid food. An enclosed sleeping area or some type of bedding is necessary for the ferret's psychological well-being. Towels, blankets, old T-shirts, sweatshirts, and the legs cut from a pair of pants work well. Occasionally, a ferret may develop the bad habit of chewing and eating cloth. This is usually a behavior of young kits and ceases to be a problem as the ferret reaches maturity. It is important to remove any torn material to decrease the opportunity for chewing. Wood or cardboard boxes with cloth lining make excellent bedding and hiding areas. Suspended hammocks and cloth tubes are also popular.

Ferrets can be litter box trained relatively easily in a cage. Place a small litter box in the corner of the cage that the pet has already selected as the toilet area. A variety of pelleted paper or other organic products may be used as litter. Clay litters (clumping or gravel) are not recommended because of the desiccating properties of this material. Ferrets are burrowing animals, and they may spend a large amount of time in the litter box with their heads and bodies buried, which can lead to a dry, brittle haircoat and upper respiratory irritation. If the pet is allowed to roam over a large area, place several litter boxes around the house, because the ferret does not always return to the cage to defecate or urinate.

With their small size and tubular body shape, ferrets can easily pass through very small openings. Exercise areas should be ferret-proofed by getting on your hands and knees and inspecting under cabinets, along baseboards, and behind appliances to make sure there are no potential holes for escape. Ferrets also burrow into furniture and mattresses and ingest foam rubber stuffing. Therefore it is advisable to cover the bottom of chairs, couches, and beds with heavy hardware cloth or wood. On more than one occasion, ferrets have met with untimely deaths by being crushed in recliner chairs where they were hiding. These chairs should be removed from the play area. Ferrets also like to hoard small items in places where they are hard to find, so it is necessary to keep clothing, shoes, keys, and other transportable items out of their reach.

It is important to select appropriate toys for ferrets. Toys that can easily be torn into small pieces are not suitable. Ferrets are attracted to all types of rubber and unfortunately tear off pieces and swallow them, resulting in gastrointestinal (GI) foreign body obstructions. Do not give ferrets soft latex rubber cat or dog toys. Keep foam rubber items such as shoes (insoles), stereo speakers, headphones, and pipe insulation out of their reach. Suitable toys include small stuffed animals (eyes and nose removed), Ping-Pong balls, golf balls, hard nylon toys, and metal balls. Ferrets enjoy running through pipes and tubes. Provide large mailing tubes, clear dryer hose, and sections of polyvinyl chloride (PVC) pipe for the pet to crawl through.

Nutrition

Mustelids are obligate carnivores, depending on a diet of small rodents, rabbits, birds, insects, reptiles, and amphibians in the wild.[2] Ferrets have a very short intestinal tract compared to dogs and cats, with a digestive transit time of 3 to 4 hours and simple gut flora.[14] In addition, they do not have a cecum or ileocolic valve, so they have a minimal ability to digest complex carbohydrates or fiber.[14] Ferrets need to eat several times a day, and it is usually best to offer food ad libitum, unless obesity is a problem. Maintenance energy requirements for ferrets are estimated as 200 to 300 kcal/kg/day, increasing to 500 kcal/kg/day for growth and reproduction.[15] Pregnancy toxemia can occur in ferrets near term if food is withheld for even 24 hours.[14] Starvation may occur inadvertently if ferrets being fed a dry diet are denied access to water (e.g., if there is a frozen water source, plugged sipper tube, or overturned water bowl).[16] Ferrets also tend to imprint on food within their first 6 months, and this lasts into adulthood. It is important for owners to feed a variety of premium ferret diets to young ferrets.

Mature pet ferrets should be fed a diet with a minimum protein level of 30 to 40%.[17] This must be in the form of high-quality meat protein with highly digestible amino acids because ferrets digest plant proteins poorly.[15] If the diet has a large amount of plant protein, particularly corn, there may be an increased risk of urolithiasis developing because of an increase in urine pH.[15] Young growing animals (up to 6 months old) and pregnant and lactating jills should receive closer to 40% high-quality protein in their diet.[16] Weaned kits receiving less than 30% dietary protein were observed to develop abnormally at Marshall Farms, a breeding facility for research beagles and ferrets (North Rose, NY).[16]

Ferrets have a high fat requirement, and the diet should contain at least 20 to 30% fat.[14,15] Ferrets frequently develop dry, brittle coats when deprived of sufficient fat in the diet.[15] Environmental factors such as low humidity or the use of clay or clumping-type litters should be ruled out. To treat a dry, brittle haircoat, use a commercially available fatty acid and give the ferret 1 to 2 cc per day. Results should be noted in 1 to 2 weeks. If there is no response, and particularly if pruritus or alopecia is present, other disease (particularly endocrine) should be investigated. Obesity is occasionally a problem in ferrets, and the amount of supplements and total volume of food will need to be controlled in these patients.

Ferrets should not be given foods that are high in refined sugars because diabetes mellitus (DM) can result.[18] Stay away from sugar-coated cereals, cakes, cookies, raisins, and other high-carbohydrate foods. Sweets can also lead to periodontal disease and can aggravate the signs of insulinoma.

Ferrets utilize fiber poorly because of their lack of intestinal flora, so diets high in fiber should be avoided.[16] Many ferrets eat fruits such as apple and melon; vegetables such as green pepper, cucumber, and potato; and cereal grains such as nonsweetened breakfast cereal or whole-grain bread. As carnivores in the wild, they eat their prey (many of them herbivores) whole and ingest the stomach contents as well. Therefore, small amounts of fruit or vegetable (not to exceed 1 teaspoon per adult ferret per day) are not harmful. Try to avoid carrots and nuts, as small pieces have caused intestinal obstruction in my experience. Also avoid raisins because of their high sugar content, particularly for ferrets suffering from insulinoma. Feeding bananas in amounts larger than 1 teaspoon has resulted in acute gastric bloat requiring surgical intervention.[18]

In Europe, Australia, and New Zealand, ferrets are fed primarily a diet of raw or cooked meat including both organ and muscle parts, with variations including the addition of dairy products, egg, meat fat, and other supplements. This type of diet more closely approximates the "natural" diet of the ferret. Whole prey items are ideal, including mice, rats, and chicks. Drawbacks of this type of diet include availability, cost, the possibility of parasite contamination, and imbalance of nutrients if only parts of the animals are fed (e.g., only muscle meat instead of organ, muscle, and bone). This "natural" diet, if it consists of fresh, parasite-free prey items, would be the most healthful for the ferret but has met with little favor in the United States. Owners can be directed to use one of the feline raw meat formulations found in sources on the subject. In the United States, the current recommendation is to feed a high-quality dry cat food or one of the specially prepared pelleted ferret foods.[14,15] Check the label to determine that the protein is primarily from a high-quality animal source and not from plant material. Ferrets generally prefer poultry and beef flavors over fish.[14] It can be difficult to change the diet once a ferret is accustomed to a particular food. Try softening the new food with warm water, using additional fat, or adding small amounts of milk to entice the ferret to eat. Because ferrets are obligate carnivores, they have difficulty utilizing carbohydrates and vegetable matter for energy, so a vegetarian diet is not recommended.[14]

Ferrets, especially those older than 2 years, can develop gastric trichobezoars. Although ferrets can vomit, they do not tend to regurgitate hairballs as frequently as cats do. Trichobezoars can reach a sufficient size to cause intestinal blockage when they are passed from the stomach. The etiology of trichobezoars in ferrets is unknown; however, it may be related to diet, lack of sufficient activity, and/or the presence of *Helicobacter mustelae* gastritis. It has been recommended in the past that approximately 1 inch of a feline hairball laxative be offered twice weekly to aid in the lubrication and removal of excess hair. Information on the efficacy of this practice is anecdotal. Be cautious about using hairball laxatives, which usually have a molasses base, in ferrets diagnosed with insulinoma.

Ferrets should be offered fresh water ad libitum. The cleanest way is to use a sipper bottle (8 to 16 ounces). If the pet is unaccustomed to drinking from a water bottle, it can become dehydrated and stop eating. This can have dire consequences, especially for kits and pregnant dams. Because ferrets like to play in water and flip the bowls over, it is best to use a heavy crock-type container. It is not necessary to add vitamins or other supplements to the water. Additives in the water can alter its taste and can enhance bacterial growth.

Reproduction

Intact males are called hobs, females are jills, and the young are called kits. A jill reaches puberty between 5 and 9 months of age, usually beginning the spring after its birth if the ferret is kept under natural lighting conditions.[4] Males reach puberty at approximately 9 months of age. Fertility may last from 2 to 5 years.[9] The females are seasonally polyestrous, from March to August, and stimulated by an increase in the photoperiod.[5] When the female is in anestrus the vulva is barely noticeable (figure 7a). When a female is in estrus, the vulva increases in size dramatically and there is a slight mucoid discharge, but no blood is present (figure 7b). Ferrets are induced ovulators, and the vulva decreases in size 1 to 2 weeks after breeding.[3] The males are sexually active from December until July in the Western Hemisphere.[3] During this time the testicles increase in size and the body and urine odors become more intense.[5] Both male and female ferrets that are "in season" may be presented with urine staining and matted fur around the perineum or abdomen. This is caused by urine being passed frequently and in small amounts for territorial marking. If urine staining is present along with dysuria, urinary tract or adrenal disease should be investigated. Surgical sterilization of male and female ferrets is recommended at 4 to 6 months of age.

Female ferrets can remain in estrus for prolonged periods of time if they are not bred, which can result in the potentially fatal condition of hyperestrogenism.[3] Hyperestrogenism can cause local or generalized alopecia or life-threatening toxic suppression of the bone marrow.[19] Bone marrow suppression and its treatment are discussed in chapter 7. The best prevention for the problems of estrus is an ovariohysterectomy (OVH) performed at 4 to 6 months of age. An OVH can be performed safely while the patient is in estrus.

Coitus in the ferret is rather active and noisy and may be shocking to the pet owner. The male ferret drags the female around by the neck and mates with her frequently. The receptive female should be submissive and, although she may cry out, she will not fight back. Wait until the female has been in estrus at least 10 days, and then place her in the male's cage for a maximum of 48 hours, or breed on 2 consecutive days. Ovulation occurs 30 to 40 hours after coitus.

During pregnancy, jills should be fed the best diet available. Food containing a minimum of 35 to 40% protein and 18 to 20% fat is adequate.[20] To prevent inadvertent fasting, do not change the diet during the pregnancy.[20] Jills that suffer a fast or carry a large litter can develop pregnancy toxemia.[3] Supplementation with high-calorie sources of nutrition is recommended if a large litter is suspected or the jill shows signs of anorexia.[20]

Fetuses can usually be palpated 2 weeks after fertilization, but palpation should not be relied on for a definitive diagnosis of pregnancy.[5] Ultrasonography can detect the fetuses at 12 days in most pregnancies.[21] Pseudopregnancy occurs if conception fails.[5] The average gestation period is 40 to 44 days (pseudopregnancies last the same amount of time).[20] A comfortable, quiet area should be set aside for whelping. A small container with a soft lining of material such as cotton batting, shredded paper, or cloth is appropriate as a whelping box.[5] Normal parturition occurs over 2 to 3 hours; any longer can indicate dystocia.[20] Kits are usually whelped by day 41 or 42 of gestation. If labor does not begin by day 43, treatment for dystocia is recommended.[20]

The litter size is 2 to 17, with 8 being average.[9] The kits are born hairless, blind, and deaf and develop a white haircoat in approximately 2 days (figure 8). In 1 week, the dark fur comes in, and by 2 to 3 weeks it is possible to tell what color the kits will be as adults (figure 9). The eyes open between 3 and 4 weeks of age (34 days average). Start feeding soft food as early as 3 weeks of age (use the adult food softened with milk or water). Kits can be weaned as early as 5 to 6 weeks of age, but it is recommended that they be left together until at least 8 weeks of age to enhance socialization.

Females return to estrus shortly after the kits are weaned unless it is late fall, in which case they will not go into estrus until the following spring if housed under natural lighting conditions.[5]

Introduction
to Medicine

Drugs and Food Supplements

Drug use and food supplementation are still in their infancy in ferret medicine. Many medications are given according to cat dosages or anecdotal information, and their efficacy and toxicity in ferrets are unknown. Dosages can also be extrapolated using allometric scaling.[22]

At this point in time, the Food and Drug Administration (FDA) has approved very few drugs for use in the ferret. Almost all such use is extra-label, and this should be explained to the owner before administration.[23] The only FDA-approved drugs labeled for use in ferrets are Imrab3 rabies vaccine (Rhone-Merieux, Athens, GA) and Fervac canine distemper vaccine (United Vaccine, Madison, WI).

Ferrets tolerate most medications well. Oral antibiotics seldom cause gastrointestinal distress. Drug administration in ferrets is similar to that in dogs and cats. For drug dosages and indications for use, see Table 3-1.

Reception, History, and Physical Examination

Ferret owners should be made aware of office visit requirements when they call to make an appointment. Receptionists should be trained in the basic health issues involved. If physically possible, a ferret should be brought to the office in the cage it lives in at home. Husbandry problems are common, and inspection of the cage can open discussion regarding proper environment, bedding, and feeding. Observe the ferret within the cage while taking the history. Obtaining a detailed history is critical to the diagnosis of disease in any ill ferret. The patient's age, gender, reproductive status, behavior, diet, environment, and signs of clinical illness should be included. In particular, note any occasions of trauma or injury and medication(s) given.

Make sure that the examination room is ferret-proof to allow observation of normal ambulation when the pet is on the floor. Place a towel or small blanket on the examining table to give the ferret traction on the slippery surface. Have the owner place the ferret on the towel; then watch carefully to prevent the ferret from falling off the table. Ferrets are very curious, and may jump without warning. Perform the physical examination as you would that of a cat or dog. Develop a routine to cover all major body systems. It is easier to do the examination piecemeal, with short breaks for the ferret to explore and relax. Minimal restraint is often more effective, and assistance is rarely needed. First, offer the ferret a non–sugar-based treat as a distraction and use a small digital thermometer to obtain a rectal temperature if necessary. Remember to weigh the patient. Gentle scruffing usually triggers the "yawn" reflex, allowing full view of the mouth and pharynx. Discuss periodontal disease at this point if tartar and/or gingivitis is found. Use an ophthalmoscope (set at black 8) to detect retinal atrophy and other ocular abnormalities. Dilate the pupil for a thorough ophthalmic examination. Check an earwax smear yearly for ear mites (*Otodectes cynotis*). Bacterial and/or yeast otitis is rare.[23] Auscultate the ferret as it is standing on the table or being scruffed. Internal organs are readily palpated in the ferret. Examine the vulva for swelling as a possible indication of estrus, retained ovary, or adrenal-associated endocrinopathy. Make owners aware of the normal vulvar dimensions in anestrus for future observation. Palpate peripheral lymph nodes for enlargement. Examine the skin and haircoat closely for alopecia, parasites, masses, and other lesions. Ferrets normally scratch vigorously, which is often mistaken as a sign of pruritus.

Preventative Health Program

Vaccine reactions occur in a small percentage of ferrets. Signs of anaphylaxis usually begin 10 minutes to several hours after vaccination.

Clinical signs include projectile vomiting, bloody diarrhea, respiratory distress, ataxia, and fever.[24,25] Anecdotally, diphenhydramine has been given for prevention and/or suppression of this response. For ferrets with no history of vaccine reaction, oral diphenhydramine (Benadryl, Parke-Davis, Morris Plains, NJ) elixir 10 to 15 minutes before a vaccine is administered has been recommended by some sources.[25] It has been suggested that any ferret with a history of vaccine reactions be pretreated with injectable diphenhydramine or corticosteroids 15 minutes before vaccination.[25] Owners should remain at the practice 30 minutes after vaccination to observe the pet for any problems. Anaphylactic reactions can occur despite pretreatment. In addition to observation at the practice, it is important that the patient be observed at home for several hours after vaccination. In the event of an anaphylactic reaction, treat with diphenhydramine, corticosteroids, epinephrine, and subcutaneous (SC) or intravenous (IV) fluids immediately.

Ferrets up to 3 years of age

The following program is recommended for the ferret patient. It is easy to follow and very useful, particularly in the older ferret, in detecting disease. The initial physical examination and consultation should be done shortly after purchase or adoption (within the guarantee period).

1. Perform a complete physical examination as already described. Include a fecal smear for detection of *Giardia* and coccidia. A fecal examination on initial presentation is suggested. Include a demonstration on ear cleaning and nail trimming. This is an excellent opportunity to discuss training, feeding, and housing. "Ferret-proofing" of the home should be stressed. Provide the name of an emergency clinic that will see ferrets after hours if your clinic does not have emergency service. Also provide information on local ferret clubs or organizations.

2. Canine distemper vaccinations should be given. At the time of this writing, Fervac-D (United Vaccine, Madison, WI) is the only distemper vaccine approved for ferrets by the U.S. Department of Agriculture (USDA). Only canine distemper vaccines of chick embryo origin should be used, as any other canine distemper vaccines, including combination vaccines, can result in clinical disease. Canine distemper vaccinations should be started at 8 weeks of age in kits from a vaccinated jill or at 4 to 6 weeks in kits from unvaccinated jills.[26] Boosters are given at 3- to 4-week intervals until the kit is a minimum of 14 weeks of age and annually thereafter.[26] Previously unvaccinated adult animals should have an initial series of two vaccinations 3 to 4 weeks apart with annual boosters thereafter.

3. Rabies vaccine is recommended for ferrets that will be around people unfamiliar with ferrets (bite potential) or at risk because of exposure to wild animals. In many states, it is required by law that all ferrets be vaccinated annually for rabies. Imrab3 (Rhone-Merieux, Athens, GA), a killed vaccine, is the only USDA-approved rabies vaccine available for ferrets at the time of this writing.[27] Give the first dose at 12 weeks of age and boosters annually thereafter. Check your local and state animal control regulations, because some agencies do not recognize the efficacy of the vaccine. In these cases, even the vaccinated ferret may be treated as a wild animal if it bites a human and must be euthanized for testing. The National Association of State Public Health Veterinarians (NASPHV) has recommended that ferrets involved in bite incidents be quarantined in the same manner as dogs and cats.[28]

4. A routine complete blood cell (CBC) count should be obtained for ferrets older than 6 months of age to screen for lymphoma. Animals younger than 6 months of age have

normally occurring lymphocytosis. Mature animals exhibit lymphocytosis primarily in the presence of chronic infection.[29] The appearance of an absolute lymphocyte count of 3500 x $10^3/\mu l$ or higher or a 60% or higher lymphocyte ratio may be an indication of early lymphoma and further diagnostics are recommended (see chapter 7).

5.   Spaying jills at 4 to 6 months of age to prevent fatal anemia should be discussed. Hobs are neutered at 4 to 8 months. Anal gland removal is not recommended as a necessary procedure. See chapter 6 for the materials and methods necessary for neutering ferrets.

6.   The client should be sent home with a hairball laxative to be given once to twice weekly during the year. Hairball laxatives may also assist in the passing of small foreign bodies but should not be used for this purpose without veterinary supervision.

7.   Heartworm prevention should be discussed and a preventative dispensed if appropriate for the geographic area. Ferrets are naturally infected with *Dirofilaria immitis*. It is difficult to detect the disease before the animal becomes ill. The CITE Snap test for heartworm antigen has proved accurate in diagnosing ferrets.[30] The American Heartworm Society recommends the use of ivermectin given orally monthly at a dose of 0.006 mg/kg. Use either the tablets for cats under 6 pounds (Heartgard, Merck, Whitehouse Station, NJ) or the injectable liquid (Ivomec, Merck, Whitehouse Station, NJ) mixed with a palatable syrup and given orally.

To summarize, annually up to 3 years of age, perform the following:

1. Complete physical examination.

2. Repeat canine distemper and rabies vaccinations.

3. Heartworm preventative if appropriate.

4. CBC count.

Ferrets older than 3 years of age

The incidence of serious disease, especially neoplasia, increases dramatically in ferrets older than 3 years of age, and early detection is the key to prolonging the pet's life in a quality manner.

1. A complete physical examination should be performed every 6 months. Carefully palpate the abdomen for splenomegaly and masses. Check all peripheral lymph nodes.

2. At least annually, a CBC count, serum biochemistries (after a 4- to 6-hour fast), and whole-body X-ray examination should be performed. These diagnostic tests can help detect insulinoma, cardiomyopathy, lymphoma, diabetes mellitus, adrenal-associated endocrinopathy, and other problems before the pet becomes critically ill. If economics are a problem for the client, a mini–geriatric testing program consisting of a CBC count and fasting blood glucose can be used for an animal that appears normal on physical examination.

3. Dental prophylaxis is performed as needed while the animal is anesthetized.

4. Annual distemper and rabies vaccines and heartworm preventative are continued.

5. Dietary adjustments should be made on the basis of any health changes detected. Ferrets older than 5 years of age should optimally have diagnostic testing and examinations performed every 6 months.

To summarize, ferrets older than 3 years of age:

1. Complete physical examination every 6 months.

2. Annual canine distemper and rabies vaccinations.

3. Heartworm preventative if appropriate.

4. CBC, blood chemistry, and whole-body X-ray examination annually (every 6 months after 5 years of age).

5. Dental prophylaxis as needed.

Table 3-1
Drugs and Dosages

Drugs and dosages listed are those most commonly used in ferrets. Dosages, applications, and duration of use may vary from case to case. Some dosages are based on empirical use and not pharmacological studies.

DRUG DOSE/ROUTE	COMMENTS
Amikacin[1] 8–16 mg/kg total per day, divided q 8–24h SC, IM, IV	If given IV, amikacin should be diluted with saline at 4 ml/kg and administered over 20 minutes to avoid neuromuscular blockade and renal failure.
Amoxicillin[1,2,*] 10–25 mg/kg q 12–24h PO, SC	May be used in combination with metronidazole and bismuth subsalicate or with only clarithromycin in the treatment of *Helicobacter mustelae* gastritis. Good broad-spectrum agent for gastrointestinal and respiratory infections.
Amoxicillin 25 mg/ml + clavulanate potassium 6.25 mg/ml[3] 12.5 mg/kg q 12h PO	
Ampicillin[4,*] 5–30 mg/kg q 12h SC, IM, IV	
Cefadroxil[*] 15–20 mg/kg q 12h PO	Broad-spectrum agent.
Cephalexin[1,*] 15–25 mg/kg q 12h PO	Broad-spectrum agent for respiratory and urinary infections.
Cephaloridine[4,*] 10–15 mg/kg q 24h SC, IM	Broad spectrum agent.
Chloramphenicol[1,2,3,*] 50 mg/kg q 12h PO (palmitate)	Chloramphenicol palmitate may be unavailable in some areas. Chloramphenicol is the treatment

NOTE: IM = intramuscularly; IV = intravenously; IT = intratracheally; PO = per os, orally; SC = subcutaneously

*Brown, S.A. Personal experience using this agent in practice situations. These listings are accompanied by pertinent comments based on anecdotal experiences.

30–50 mg/kg q 12h SC, IM, IV
(succinate)

of choice for proliferative bowel disease. Use for a
minimum of 14 days. Advise owner of potential
human toxicities from contact.

Ciprofloxacin[1,2,3,*]
5–15 mg/kg q 12h PO or
10–30 mg/kg q 24h PO

Used in the same situations as enrofloxacin.

**Ciprofloxacin hydrochloride
0.3% ophthalmic**[3]
2–3 drops q 12h topically

Clarithromycin[*]
50 mg/kg q 12–24h PO

Use in combination with amoxicillin or
metronidazole plus bismuth subsalicylate for
the treatment of *Helicobacter mustelae* gastritis.

Clindamycin hydrochloride[3,*]
5.5–10 mg/kg q 12h PO

For anaerobic infections. Good for bone and dental
disease.

Cloxacillin[1,2,3]
10 mg/kg q 6h PO, IM, IV

Enrofloxacin[1,3,*]
5–10 mg/kg q 12h PO, SC, IM,
or 10–20 mg/kg q 24h PO,
SC, IM

Broad-spectrum agent; however, this drug has been
overused and antibiotic resistance may ultimately
be the result in the future. May use IM for a few
days, but sterile abscesses may result. Oral
administration is preferred. Injectable form may
be mixed with a palatable syrup.

Erythromycin[1,2,3]
10–15 mg/kg q 6h PO

Gentamicin[1,2,3]
1–8 mg/kg total per day,
divided q 8–24h SC, IM, IV

If given IV, gentamicin should be diluted with saline
at 4 ml/kg and administered over 20 minutes to avoid
neuromuscular blockade and renal failure.

Lincomycin[1,2]
10–15 mg/kg q 8h PO or
10 mg/kg q 12h IM

continued

Metronidazole[1,*]
10–25 mg/kg *q* 12h PO

For anaerobic infections. May be used along with
amoxicillin or clarithromycin in the treatment
of *Helicobacter mustelae* gastritis. May be used
along with chloramphenicol for proliferative colitis.

Neomycin[1,2,3]
10–20 mg/kg *q* 6–12h PO

Netilmicin[1]
6–8 mg/kg *q* 24h SC, IM, IV

If given IV, netilmicin should be diluted with saline
at 4 ml/kg and administered over 20 minutes
to avoid neuromuscular blockade and renal
failure.

Oxytetracycline[1,2]
20 mg/kg *q* 8h PO

**Penicillin G
(sodium or potassium)**[1,2,*]
40,000 IU/kg *q* 24h IM or
  20,000 IU/kg *q* 12h IM

Sulfadimethoxine[1,3,*]
25 mg/kg *q* 24h PO, SC, IM

Sulfasoxazole[3]
50 mg/kg *q* 8h PO

Tetracycline[1,3]
25 mg/kg *q* 8–12h PO

**Trimethoprim–sulfa
combinations**[1,3,4,*]
15–30 mg/kg *q* 12h PO, SC

Dose is based on the mg amount of *combined* drugs.

Tylosin[1,2,*]
10 mg/kg *q* 12–24h PO

ANTIPARASITIC AGENTS

Amitraz[1]

Apply to affected skin 3–6 times at 14-day intervals.

Amprolium[4]
19 mg/kg *q* 24h PO

Carbaryl[1,*]
0.5% shampoo or 5% powder   Treat once a week for 3–6 weeks.

Decoquinate[4]
0.5 mg/kg *q* 24h PO   Mix in moist food.

Diethylcarbamazine[2,3]
2.75–11 mg/kg *q* 24h PO   Heartworm preventative; ivermectin is preferred.

Imidacloprid[*]
0.4 ml/ferret of 9.1% solution   For flea control. Appears to be safe.
  q 30d topically

Ivermectin[1,2,*]
0.006 mg/kg *q* 30d PO   For heartworm prevention. Can use canine
    products.

0.5 mg/kg PO, SC   Heartworm microfilaricide; 3–4 week post-
    adulticide treatment.

0.50–1.0 mg/kg PO, SC   Use at this dosage range for sarcoptic mange.
    Repeat at 2-week intervals for at least three
    doses.
    For *Otodectes* infestation use 1.0 mg/kg dose, putting
    one half of the total dose in each ear; repeat
    in 2 weeks.

Lime sulfur[1]

    Dilute 1:40 in water; wash ferret with solution
    once a week for 6 weeks.

Luferon[*]
30 mg/kg *q* 30d PO   For flea control. Appears to be safe in ferrets.

Metronidazole
20 mg/kg *q* 12–24h PO[1,3,*]   For gastrointestinal protozoal infections. Use for
  or 35 mg/kg *q* 24h PO[2,*]   5 to 10 days.

Milbemycin oxime[1,3,*]
1.15–2.33 mg/kg *q* 30d PO   Use for heartworm prevention. Use smallest
    dose canine tablets.

Piperazine[1,3]
50–100 mg/kg *q* 14d PO   Use at least two doses.

continued

Praziquantel[1,2,*]
5–12.5 mg/ferret PO, SC;
  repeat in14 days

Use for cestodes.

Pyrantel pamoate[2,3]
4.4 mg/kg PO;
  repeat in 14 days

Pyrethrin products[1,*]

Use topically as directed once per week as needed.

Sulfadimethoxine[1,*]
50 mg/kg PO once; then
  25 mg/kg q 24h for 9 days
  PO

For coccidial infections.

ANTIFUNGAL AGENTS

Amphotericin B[1,3]
0.4–0.8 mg/kg *q* 7d IV

Total dose not to exceed 25 mg, or follow
  published canine protocols.

Griseofulvin[1,3]
25 mg/kg *q* 24h PO

Follow feline protocols.

Ketoconazole[1,2,3]
10–50 mg/kg *q* 12–24h PO

Not effective for controlling signs of adrenal
  disease.

MISCELLANEOUS AGENTS

Amantidine
6 mg/kg *q* 12h PO

Antiviral agent. May be useful in the treatment
  of influenza in ferrets.

Aminophylline[1,*]
4 mg/kg *q* 12h PO, IM, IV

Bronchodilation.

Atenolol[5]
6.25 mg/ferret *q* 24h PO

Beta-adrenergic blocker used in hypertrophic
  cardiomyopathy.

Atropine sulfate[1,3]
5–10 mg/kg SC, IM

For organophosphate toxicity. See anesthetic section for dose as preanesthetic.

Barium (20%)[*]
15 mg/kg PO

Used for gastrointestinal contrast study.

Bismuth subsalicylate[1,*]
0.25 mg/kg *q* 8–12h PO

Used in conjunction with other drugs for treatment of gastric ulcers. Ferrets object to its tase, so it may have to be mixed with a palatable syrup.

Captopril[2]
1.6 mg/kg (1/8 of tablet) *q* 48h PO

Vasodilator. This is the starting dose. Eventually, increase frequency to *q* 12–24h. Can cause lethargy.

Chlorpheniramine[*]
1–2 mg/kg *q* 8–12h PO

Antihistamine for control of sneezing and coughing.

Cimetidine[1,2,*]
5–10 mg/kg *q* 8h PO, SC, IM, IV

Inhibits gastric acid secretion. Used for treatment of gastric ulcers. Unpalatable; should be mixed with a palatable syrup. Give IV bolus slowly.

Cisapride[1,3]
0.5 mg/kg *q* 8h PO

Gastrointestinal mobility stimulant.

Dexamethasone[*]
0.5–2.0 mg/kg PO, SC, IM, IV

Dexamethasone sodium phosphate[1,*]
4–8 mg/kg IM, IV, once

Use for initial shock therapy.

Diazoxide[1,2,*]
5–30 mg/kg *q* 12h PO

Insulin-blocking agent used in the treatment of insulinoma. Start at the low end of the dose and gradually work up to effective dose. Usually used in conjunction with corticosteroids. May cause hypertension, lethargy, depression, and/or nausea.

continued

Digoxin elixir[1,2,3,*]
0.005–0.01 mg/kg *q* 12–24h
PO for maintenance

Positive inotrope for dilated cardiomyopathy. Start with higher dose to load for the first 24–48 hours, then reduce. Monitor blood digoxin concentration if possible.

Diltiazem[1,5]
1.5–7.5 mg/kg *q* 12h PO

Calcium channel blocker used for hypertrophic cardiomyopathy. Adjust dose as needed.

Diphenhydramine[1,*]
0.5–2 mg/kg *q* 8–12h PO, IM

Antihistamine used to control sneezing and coughing. Useful in treating anaphylactic reactions to vaccination. May be used prevaccination in cases where previous anaphylaxis occurred. However, note that this pretreatment may not be 100% effective.

Doxapram[1,2,3,6]
1–11 mg/kg IV

Respiratory stimulant.

Enalapril[1,3,5,*]
0.25–0.5 mg/kg *q* 24–48h PO

Vasodilator for dilated cardiomyopathy. Well tolerated. Monitor for weakness and anorexia. Use with caution when renal disease is present.

Enteral feeding[3]
200–300 kcal/day

This is maintenance level. Best to give assist feedings in 4–6 small meals a day.

Epinephrine
20 mcg/kg SC, IM, IV, IT

Used for treating anaphylactic reactions.

Epoetin alpha[*]
50–150 IU/kg *q* 48h PO, IM

50–150 IU/kg *q* 7d PO, IM, for maintenance

Useful in stimulating red blood cell production (chemotherapy, renal disease, etc.). Use *q* 48h until desired pack cell volume is reached and then use maintenance dose.

Famotidine[*]
0.25–0.50 mg/kg *q* 24h PO, IV

Inhibits gastric acid secretion. Used in gastric ulcer therapy.

Filigrastim[*]
5 mg/kg *q* 24h SC

A human granulocyte colony stimulating factor. Used in chemotherapy.

Fluid therapy[3,*]
60–75 ml/kg q 24h PO, SC, IV

This is maintenance fluid level. Be sure to correct for dehydration.

Flurbiprofen sodium[3]
1–2 drops *q* 12–24h topically

Topical NSAID for ophthalmic inflammation.

Flutamide[7]
10 mg/kg *q* 12h PO

Antiandrogenic drug used to alleviate the signs of adrenal neoplasia or hyperplasia. Most useful for reducing enlarged periurethral tissue. Lifetime treatment. Tablets can be made into a pleasant tasting suspension.

Furosemide[5,*]
1–4 mg/kg *q* 8–12h PO, SC, IM, IV

Diuretic. First drug commonly used in treating cardiac disease.

GnRH[2,*]
20 mcg/ferret once, IM

Used to terminate estrus. Give after ferret has been in estrus for a minimum of 10 days. Repeat in 14 days if no response. Perform complete blood cell count to detect anemia if ferret has been in estrus 21 days or longer.

hCG[1,2,3,*]
100 IU/ferret once, IM

Used to terminate estrus. Same directions apply as for GnRH.

Hydrocortisone sodium succinate[2,3]
25–40 mg/kg IV

For shock therapy.

Hydroxyzine hydrochloride[1]
2 mg/kg *q* 8h PO

Used for management of some types of pruritis. Because it acts as a mild sedative, it should be used with great caution with central nervous system depressant drugs. May cause drowsiness.

continued

Insulin, NPH[2],*

0.5–6.0 IU/kg *q* 12–24h
or to effect, SC

Used for treatment of diabetes mellitus and other hyperglycemic conditions (e.g., glucagonoma or postsurgically after insulinoma removal). Follow similar guidelines as for the feline patient. Other forms of insulin may be tried. Oral hypoglycemics do not appear to be effective in ferrets.

Iron dextran[1,3]

10 mg/ferret IM

Kaolin/pectin[1],*

1–2 ml/kg *q* 2–6h as needed, PO   Gastrointestinal coating agent.

Lactulose syrup[1],*

1.5–3 mg/kg *q* 12h PO

Absorbs blood ammonia (as in hepatic disease). May cause soft stools at higher dose due to its laxative effect.

Loperamide*

0.2 mg/kg *q* 12h PO

Anitidiarrheal. Useful in the treatment of epizootic catarrhal gastroenteritis (ECE).

Melarsamine hydrochloride

2.5 mg/kg IM once, followed
1 month later by two doses
IM 24 hours apart

Used for treatment of heartworm disease.

Metoclopramide[1]

0.2–1 mg/kg *q* 6–8h PO, SC   Gastrointestinal motility stimulant.

Mitotane (o,p'–DDD)*

50 mg/ferret *q* 24h for 7 days;
then *q* 48h until signs
resolved; then *q* 7d or
as needed

Chemotherapy drug specific for adrenal tissue. Used to treat adrenocortical neoplasia or hyperplasia. Drug should be placed into small gelatin capsules by a pharmacist. Results are variable; drug may alleviate signs for a period of time but rarely results in a cure.

Nitroglycerine 2% Ointment[2,3]

1/16–1/8 inch/ferret *q* 12–24h
topically on shaved inner
thigh or pinna

Vasodilator for cardiomyopathy.

Oxytocin[1,2,*]

0.2–10 USP units/kg SC, IM   Expels retained fetus and stimulates lactation.

Prednisone, prednisolone[1,2,3,*]

0.10–2.5 mg/kg q 12–24h PO   Corticosteriod with multiple uses (chemotherapy, insulinoma, eosinophilic gastroenteritis, etc.). When treating early insulinoma, start with lowest dose q 12h and increase as needed to control signs.

Prochlorperazine[3]

0.13 mg/kg q 3–4h deep IM   For control of nausea and vomiting.

Proligestone[1]

50 mg/kg once, IM   Use before onset of female reproductive season.

Propanolol[1,2,*]

0.50–2.0 mg/kg q 12–24h PO, SC   Beta blocker and vasodilator used in hypertrophic cardiomyopathy. May cause lethargy and anorexia.

Prostaglandin F2 alpha

0.1–0.5 mg/ferret as needed, IM   Used in metritis to help expel necrotic debris.

Stanozolol[1,3,*]

0.5 mg/kg q 24h PO, SC, IM, or 10–25 mg/kg q 7d PO, SC, IM   Anabolic steroid.

Sucralfate[1,3,*]

25 mg/kg up to 125 mg/ferret q 6–8h PO   Used in treatment of gastrointestinal ulcers. Do not use with cimetidine or other antacids as sucralfate is active only in an acid environment.

Sulfasalazine[1]

10–20 mg/kg q 12h PO   Used in treatment of ulcerative enteritis or colitis.

Theophylline elixir[1,3,*]

4.25 mg/kg q 8–12h PO   Bronchodilator.

Vitamin B complex[1,*]

1–2 mg/kg as needed, IM   Dose listed is based on thiamine content.

References

1. Smith, D.A., and Burgman, P.M. Formulary. In Hillyer, E.V., and Quesenberry, K.E., eds., Ferrets, rabbits and rodents: Clinical medicine and surgery, pp. 394–397. Philadelphia: W.B. Saunders; 1997.

2. Carpenter, J.W., Mashima, T.Y., and Rupiper, D.J. Exotic animal formulary. Manhattan, KS: Greystone; 1996.

3. Johnson-Delaney, C.A. Exotic companion medicine handbood. Lake Worth, FL: Wingers Publishing.

4. Hawk, D.F., and Leary, S.L. Formulary for laboratory animals. Ames: Iowa State Press; 1995.

5. Stamoulis, M.E. Cardiac diesease in ferrets. Sem Avian Exotic Pet Med 4:43–48; 1995.

6. Flecknell, P.A. Laboratory animal anesthesia. London: Academic Press; 1987.

7. Rosenthal, K.R. Personal communication; 1997.

Clinical Techniques

Oral Medication

It can be difficult to administer a pill to a ferret, so other alternatives are encouraged. Oral medications can be given in suspension with sweet or oily liquid from a syringe or crushed and mixed with a palatable substance, such as baby food or fatty acid supplement. Because of the small amount needed, it is very helpful to have medications compounded by a licensed compounding pharmacy. For many medications, a good relationship with a compounding pharmacy for sweet (but sugar-free) or meat-flavored liquids is essential. Local pharmacies can often provide suspensions as well and at less expense but are usually limited to fruit flavors.

A syringe is used to administer liquid medications. The ferret is scruffed and held upright, with the hind limbs touching the table or your lap. As the ferret yawns, place the tip of the syringe caudal to the lower canine teeth and slowly drip the medication into the mouth.

Alternatively, the ferret can be given medication while restrained in dorsal recumbency, its head in the palm of your hand and the body held by your forearm against your side. To administer a pill, place the index finger and thumb of the restraining hand behind the upper canine teeth and apply pressure until the ferret opens its mouth. Drop the pill into the back of the mouth and use a finger or a soft-tipped object (such as the eraser end of a pencil) to push the pill over the back of the tongue. A cat pill gun can also be used. Immediately after administration, offer a pleasant-tasting liquid such as strained-meat baby food diluted with water to aid swallowing.[12]

Postoperative patients and debilitated animals often need assisted feeding. Most will lap high-protein and fat combinations from a syringe or spoon, but a few will need assisted feeding or tube feeding if completely anorectic. The caloric maintenance requirement for the ferret is 200 to 300 Kc/kg per 24 hours. Liquid diets used for ferrets must contain a high percentage of protein and fat. A liquid diet should be fed in a volume no larger than 20 cc per ferret per feeding three to six times daily.[12] A variety of products are currently used to provide liquid nutrition to the ferret, including Deliver 2.0 (Mead Johnson Nutritionals, Evansville, IN) and Ensure Plus and Sustacal (Abbott Laboratories, Columbus, OH). These are often blenderized with strained-meat baby food, a/d (Hill's Pet Products, Topeka, KS), or beef liver and warmed before administration.

Injectable Medication

Give subcutaneous (SC) injections between the shoulder blades or along the neck. Scruff the ferret to make these areas accessible and as an effective restraint. The ferret may be offered a treat while injecting to provide a distraction. Do not use sugar-based treats if a fasting glucose test is needed. The skin is quite thick and tough, and a small-gauge needle (23–27 gauge) penetrates most easily. Placing a small amount of a treat on a tongue depressor in front of the ferret is generally all the restraint necessary beforehand.

Give intramuscular (IM) injections into the lumbar or quadriceps muscles. The SC route is preferred in this species because of the lack of muscle mass. Lumbar or caudal thigh muscles accommodate small volumes injected with a 25- to 27-gauge needle. The patient should be scruffed and may be distracted with a treat.

Blood Collection

Phlebotomy procedures in ferrets are similar to those in cats. Blood volume in ferrets is approximately 7 to 10% of body weight, and 10% of this volume can be taken safely.[32] For example, a healthy 1000-g ferret could safely lose 7 to 10 cc of blood. Use small collection containers and remove the needle from the syringe before transferring the blood to avoid hemolysis. Do not use tubes with large quantities of liquid anticoagulant because this will dilute the sample. Use small-gauge needles (25–27) for venipuncture attached to an insulin or tuberculin (TB) syringe to avoid collapsing the vein. For larger samples, use up to a 22-gauge needle with a 6-cc syringe via the jugular vein or vena cava.

Sedation is seldom necessary once you have gained some experience. Ferrets often struggle vigorously and defecate and urinate when first restrained for blood collection. After a short struggle, the patient usually becomes calm and tolerates phlebotomy.[12] If treats are used, avoid sugar if an accurate blood glucose test is needed. If sedation is necessary, isoflurane can be used, but has been shown to decrease hematologic values artificially, particularly packed cell volume (PCV), red blood cell (RBC) count, and white blood cell (WBC) count.[33] Medetomidine (Domitor, Orion Corporation, Espoo, Finland) is a good choice for fast induction and is quickly reversed with atipamezole (Antisedan, Orion Corporation, Espoo, Finland).[34] It is rarely necessary to clip hair from the venipuncture site once proficiency with phlebotomy is acquired. Discuss shaving of the coat with the owner beforehand, as hair regrowth can take 1 to 3 months.

Avoid toenail clipping as a method of blood collection. It is painful to the ferret, and the sample can be contaminated with tissue fluids.

To obtain small amounts of blood, use a 25-gauge needle with a 0.5- to 1-cc syringe in the cephalic or saphenous (medial or lateral) veins or the tail artery. To use the cephalic (figure 10) or saphenous veins (figure 11), have the handler scruff the ferret or grasp it firmly around the neck with one hand while holding off the vein or extending the leg with the other (similar to the procedure used with a cat).[12] A tourniquet may facilitate vein location but is not tolerated by many ferrets. When blood is aspirated into the syringe, release pressure on the vein to allow the blood to flow. Alternatively, place the needle in the vein without a syringe attached and allow blood to flow directly into the collection tube.

The tail artery is the last choice for a blood collection site because it is painful to the patient and hemolysis of the sample is more likely. Either have the handler scruff the ferret or wrap it securely in a towel to minimize movement.[12] Insert a 22- or 25-gauge needle at a 60 to 90° angle 2 to 5 cm from the tail base into the ventral aspect. Insert the needle until it touches the ventral surface of the vertebrae, then slowly retract the needle while gently aspirating until blood is drawn. Up to 1 to 3 ml can be drawn from this site.[35]

The jugular vein is used to collect larger amounts of blood (figure 12). There are several techniques for jugular blood collection. The first is similar to that used in the cat. Use a 20- to 22-gauge needle with a 3-cc or larger syringe. Extend the ferret's neck and pull the forelegs downward over the edge of the table, with the ferret's body held closely to the handler with her or his elbow and forearm. Apply pressure just lateral to the thoracic inlet, and visualize and/or palpate the jugular vessel running laterally on a line from the thoracic inlet to the base of the ear. Insert the needle at a shallow angle. The most common mistake is to probe too deeply for the vein. It can be helpful to bend the needle at a slight angle. The presence of subcutaneous fat, particularly in the intact male, can make the vein difficult to visualize.

A second method of jugular venipuncture is as follows. Scruff the ferret and suspend the animal over a table. Wrap the body in a towel at the level of the thoracic inlet, folding the forelimbs caudally (figure 13a). Have the handler scruff the ferret just along the cranial half of the neck and place the patient in dorsal recumbency. Apply pressure lateral to the thoracic inlet and draw the blood as described in the preceding method (figure 13b).

A third method can be used for some ferrets with no assistance. Place the ferret in ventral recumbency on the table. Extend its neck with one hand by placing the index finger under the chin and the thumb across the thoracic inlet. Wrap the rest of the fingers of this hand around the ferret's neck. Use little or no restraint on the body. When the ferret is calm, usually after a brief struggle, access the vein as previously described.[12]

The cranial vena cava can also be used when large amounts of blood are needed, but this can be done only with a sedated or extremely well-restrained animal to avoid laceration of the vessel. Do not attempt this procedure if intrathoracic disease is suspected. With two handlers, grasp the ferret firmly and hold in dorsal recumbency, extend the neck in a horizontal position, pull the forelegs caudally, and restrain the hind limbs. Use a 25-gauge needle and a 3-cc syringe, and insert the needle through the skin in the notch between the manubrium and the first rib. Aim the needle toward the opposite hip at a shallow angle. Move the needle slowly caudally with gentle suction until blood enters the hub, and draw the sample. Because this is a blind technique, the potential for complications exists, especially if insufficient restraint is used.[13]

Blood Transfusion

Ferrets have no apparent blood types; therefore any healthy ferret can be a donor without typing or cross-matching.[36] Blood volume in ferrets is 7 to 10% of their body weight.[32] In healthy animals, it is safe to remove 10 to 20% of this volume.[37] For example, a 1000-g ferret would have a blood volume of 70 to 100 cc, and it would be safe to remove 7 to 20 cc of blood every 21 days.[37] All donors should be screened for Aleutian disease and heartworm.[38] Although it has not been proved that lymphoma is contagious, screening via a complete blood cell (CBC) count is recommended. Transfusion is indicated in cases of blood loss, estrogen toxicity, and anemia of chronic disease when the PCV is less than 15%.[32] Flush a 20- to 23-gauge butterfly catheter with acid-citrate-dextrose (ACD) anticoagulant solution.[37] The jugular vein or cranial vena cava should be used because of the large volume of blood required. Sedation is used if necessary. Draw the blood directly into a syringe with 1 cc of ACD per 6 cc collected.[37] Dilute heparin can also be used.[18] Treat the recipient with one dose of a fast-acting intravenous (IV) corticosteroid, such as dexamethasone sodium phosphate (4–8 mg/kg) or prednisolone sodium succinate (2.5

mg/kg).[37] Administer the blood immediately into the recipient via a butterfly catheter or already indwelling IV or intraosseous (IO) catheter. Interperitoneal administration of blood is acceptable if a venous route is unavailable.[37]

Catheters

IV catheters can be placed in the cephalic, jugular, or lateral saphenous veins. A short, small-gauge (22–25 gauge), over-the-needle catheter works well. Use standard sterile catheter preparation of the area. In most patients, especially the severely dehydrated, it is necessary to nick the skin with a 20- to 22-gauge needle or No. 15 blade to facilitate catheter placement. Use 0.5-inch adhesive or paper tape to secure the catheter. Cover the catheter cap with two or three layers of bandage material. A bitter substance on the bandages will also deter chewing.

Intraosseous (IO) catheters are a reasonable alternative when the IV route is unavailable. This option is especially useful for severely dehydrated or vein-damaged patients. Anesthesia is necessary in most patients. The femur is the most common site for IO catheter placement, but the humerus and tibia can also be used.[39] Surgically prepare the area over the femoral head. Make a small skin incision over the greater trochanter. A spinal needle (20–22 gauge, 1.5 inch) is preferred because of the stylet to prevent bone plugs and the superior strength of the needle. However, a 20- to 22-gauge, 1- to 1.5-inch hypodermic needle may also be used, with a sterile 30-gauge surgical wire stylet. Insert a hypodermic needle or spinal needle medial to the greater trochanter into the marrow cavity using firm pressure and gentle rotation.[39] Remove the stylet and place a tape butterfly on the hub of the needle and suture it to the skin (figure 14). Fluids and other medications (except chemotherapy agents) normally given intravenously can be given by slow drip directly into the marrow cavity. IO catheters can remain in place for 48 to 72 hours. The catheter should be removed when the ferret becomes more active to prevent ending of the needle. Broad-spectrum antibiotics should be administered for the duration of catheter placement and for 1 week thereafter.

Bone Marrow Biopsy

Bone marrow biopsy is an excellent diagnostic aid for ferrets exhibiting nonregenerative anemia, pancytopenia, thrombocytopenia, and other hematologic abnormalities. In addition, bone marrow evaluation is critical in determining appropriate chemotherapy. Aspiration is the method of choice. Bone marrow sampling can be done using the long bones or pelvis.

A technique has been described for femoral bone marrow collection.[40] Place the anesthetized patient in lateral recumbency and prepare the proximal femur aseptically. Palpate the greater trochanter as a landmark, and make a stab incision with a No. 15 blade through the skin.[40] Position a spinal needle (20 gauge, 1.5 inch) to the greater trochanter while holding the hind limb firmly with the other hand.[40] Insert the needle into the bone with steady pressure and an alternating rotating motion.[40] When the needle is firmly embedded in the marrow cavity, remove the stylet and attach a 10-cc syringe to suction marrow fluid into the syringe.[40] Stop the suction as soon as the fluid reaches the syringe to prevent blood contamination.[40] Remove the needle and prepare bone marrow smears for examination.[40]

Urine Collection

A urinalysis should be performed in suspected cases of urogenital disease, metabolic disease, and trauma. Urine is collected via free catch, manual expression of the bladder, catheterization, or cystocentesis. Owners can provide samples collected from a litter box prepared by emptying the litter but not antiseptically cleaning the box so as to retain the odor of urine.[12] Nonabsorbable pellets or beads (Nosorb, Catco Inc., Tiffen, OH) can be used in place of litter if necessary to collect a sample. The normal ferret bladder is small but resistant to rupture under firm pressure. Manual expression of urine is possible with most animals.

Urine can also be collected via catheterization, although this can be difficult because of the small size of the urethral opening and complicated in the male by the J-shaped os penis. Unfortunately, it is often necessary due to partial or total obstruction of the urethra by cystic calculi or enlarged prostatic tissue. Catheterization allows a clean sample for urinalysis and a passage for contrast materials during radiographic studies.[12] A variety of materials are utilized as catheters in ferrets, including open- or closed-end tom cat catheters, jugular or IV catheters, and 3.5 French feeding tubes. Flexible tubing may require a stylet.[12] There is now a 3.0 French urinary catheter designed specifically for ferrets (Cook Veterinary Products Inc., Bloomington, IN). Storage of flexible tubes in the freezer decreases the need for a stylet. Lubricate the entire length of the catheter before use.

For female ferrets, elevate the hindquarters of the anesthetized patient with a rolled towel beneath the abdomen while it is in ventral recumbency.[41] Surgically prepare the vulva and perivulvar area. Use an otoscope to visualize the blind clitoral fossa on the ventral floor of the vestibule immediately cranial to the mucocutaneous junction.[41] The urethral orifice is located 1 to 1.5 cm cranial to the fossa.[41] Pass the catheter into this opening.

Place anesthetized male ferrets in dorsal recumbency and aseptically prepare the skin around the prepuce. Diazepam administration relaxes smooth muscles before catheter placement.[42] Exteriorize the distal end of the penis to locate the urethral orifice on the ventral surface.[41] Urine expression may be necessary for proper visualization.[41] If the preputial opening is too small, make a small incision to enlarge the opening and allow the penis to be extended.[12] A fine-tipped forceps can be used to enter gently and spread the urethral opening for catheter insertion.[12] In cases of resistance to catheterization, a syringe filled with warm saline attached to the catheter to introduce small volumes of fluid will dilate the urethra to allow passage.[12] Lidocaine can be infused into the urethra to aid catheter placement.[42] The catheter can be sutured in place to allow urination in the presence of a blockage, but this is not tolerated well by ferrets. The catheter and any small parts can become gastrointestinal foreign bodies in the active patient.[12]

Cystocentesis provides a clean sample for bacterial culture and sensitivity and provides relief for the obstructed patient. Anesthesia is recommended for all but the most depressed patients, as movement can lead to laceration of the bladder by the needle.[12]

Urine culture specimens should be incubated in sterile culture containers at room temperature for 1 hour before refrigeration to improve culture yields.

Tissue Biopsies

Popliteal nodectomy

Biopsy is recommended in cases of generalized lymphadenopathy or peripheral lymphocytosis to determine the presence of lymphoma. A needle aspirate of most lymph nodes is nearly impossible because of the large amount of perinodal fat. Superficial nodes available for removal include the axillary, prescapular, popliteal, and inguinal.[12] The popliteal lymph node lies in a pocket of subcutaneous fat proximal to the stifle on the caudal thigh and is the most accessible.

Place the anesthetized ferret in ventral recumbency. Surgically prepare the posterior aspect of the thigh. Grasp the muscle mass on the posterior aspect of the thigh and palpate a firm movable mass in the midthigh, which represents the lymph node and the perinodal fat.[12] Grasp the node and pull it toward the skin (in much the same way as one would stabilize a testicle through the scrotum during a castration).[12] Make a small incision through the skin over this area, and the fat will protrude.[12] Gently dissect through the fat while firmly holding behind the mass.[12] Avoid aggressive fat removal, which increases bleeding. Dissect free the tan lymph node when it is visualized.[12] No ligation is necessary. Surrounding blood vessels are easily avoided.[12]

Close the skin with subcuticular or skin sutures.[12] Remove sutures in 7 to 10 days. Recovery from this procedure is usually unremarkable; however, a few ferrets will chew the sutures if they are too tight or if deep or aggressive dissection was performed.[12]

Splenic aspirate

Splenomegaly is a common clinical finding in the ferret. Although it is usually a benign condition, it may be necessary to rule out the presence of splenic disease. A percutaneous splenic aspirate provides appropriate material for cytology.

Sedation is seldom necessary. Aseptically prepare an area of the skin where the spleen is easily accessible to the left lateral and ventral body wall.[12] Restrain the ferret in dorsal recumbency. Grasp the spleen and hold it firmly against the body wall.[12] Use a 25-gauge needle attached to a 3-cc syringe and apply vigorous suction to aspirate a small amount of bloody fluid for cytology.[12]

Splenic biopsy

Splenic biopsy is indicated when abdominal exploration reveals abnormalities. For a sample of the margin, place mattress sutures through both surfaces of the spleen.[42] Transect the parenchyma distal to the sutures, leaving them in place to control hemorrhage.[42] To remove a central portion of the spleen, make two parallel incisions long and deep enough for a representative sample.[42] Make two additional incisions perpendicular to the original incisions to remove a rectangle of tissue.[42] Place mattress sutures across the defect to control hemorrhage.[42]

Tracheal Wash

The procedure is the same as that performed in the cat. Place a sterile endotracheal tube after general anesthetic induction. Use a sterile catheter to introduce 1 to 3 cc of sterile saline into the bronchiolar tree. Immediately aspirate as much fluid as possible and remove the catheter. Perform culture and cytology on the aspirated fluid as needed.

Radiography

Use high-detail radiographic techniques for ferrets, with high-resolution film-screen combinations, a short exposure time (less than /60 second), a high mA, and a kVp of approximately 50.[43] A grid is not needed. Position the patient directly on the plate.[43] A dental X-ray unit is useful for skull and oral X rays. Full-body radiographs are recommended on initial presentation, with later detail films taken as needed.[44] Awake ferrets can be restrained using an orange IV line clamp firmly fastened in the scruff, with small sandbags, foam pads, and/or tape for positioning. Use isoflurane sedation to obtain diagnostic films and prevent radiation exposure of the humans involved.[44] Changes in the cardiac silhouette, thoracic masses (particularly mediastinal), and organomegaly are readily visualized in this fashion. In my experience, ferrets older than 4 years often have enlarged heart silhouettes on routine radiographs without evidence of clinical disease on electrocardiography or ultrasonography. These animals should be followed closely thereafter for the onset of disease. Radiographs are not usually diagnostic for either adrenal gland enlargement or insulinoma, because of the small organs involved.

Myelography

Myelography is a useful technique for determining the site of spinal trauma or neoplasia. Both cerebrospinal fluid spinal taps and myelography can be performed at the atlanto-occipital and lumbar (L5–L6) regions. Use a 20- to 22-gauge spinal needle as described for cats and dogs.[45] Iohexol is an appropriate contrast medium (0.25–0.05 ml/kg). Treatment with prednisolone sodium succinate (30 mg/kg IV once) may prevent seizures and edema.[45]

Electrocardiography

An electrocardiogram (ECG) is important for detecting arrhythmias and conduction abnormalities in the ferret.[31] Unfortunately, the patient is seldom cooperative. Use flattened or padded alligator clips for the patient's comfort, or sedate with isoflurane.[44] Ferrets with cardiac abnormalities can present with sinus rhythm or tachycardia, first- or second-degree heart block, and/or premature ventricular or atrial contractions.[31,44] Use the information from the ECG in conjunction with further diagnostic methods such as ultrasonography for a complete diagnosis.

Ultrasonography

Ultrasonography is used with increasing frequency with ferrets as a diagnostic tool. It is helpful in pregnancy diagnosis, as embryonic vesicles are detectable by real-time ultrasonographic imaging at 12 days.[21] Ultrasonography is frequently recommended as a diagnostic aid in adrenal disease. Unfortunately, one study suggested that abnormalities of the adrenal glands themselves are found in only approximately 50% of positive cases.[46] However, ultrasonography can be useful in detecting paraurethral cysts in male ferrets with adrenal disease. Ultrasonography is valuable in detecting abdominal neoplasia, hepatic disease, renal disease, lymph node enlargement, and cardiac and thoracic abnormalities.[46] It is the most accurate method for diagnosing cardiac disease in the ferret.[47]

5

Anesthesia

Introduction

Anesthesia for ferrets is an active field of research. Because of the ferret's increased presence in both research and clinical practice, access to quick, safe anesthesia and efficacious analgesia is a necessity. The basic precautions are similar to those used with other companion animals: monitoring of cardiopulmonary stability and maintaining hydration and body temperature before, during, and after any general anesthesia exposure.[48] Also, differences in anesthetic susceptibility related to age, gender, overall health, and environment must be considered. It is useful to have emergency drugs prepared before any anesthetic procedure involving a high-risk patient.

All patients prepared for anesthesia should be assessed for respiratory and cardiac disease. Subclinical cardiac disease can be a fatal complication in procedures involving general anesthesia and surgery.[49] Food should be withheld 4 to 6 hours before anesthetic induction.[11] Fasting for longer periods can result in severe hypoglycemia.[49] Remove water 1 hour before anesthetic induction. Ferrets seldom vomit with anesthesia, but they should be monitored accordingly. Thermoregulation does not return until full recovery; therefore, monitor body temperature and use a warm-water–circulating heating pad and warmed towels or an incubator postoperatively. Be aware that hyperthermia can occur quickly if the patient is not watched closely during this period.

Anesthetic Options

Isoflurane is the anesthetic of choice for most procedures in ferret medicine.[11] It has proved to be very safe for even the most critical patient.[50] Isoflurane can be used for outpatient procedures such as blood collection or radiography. Note that isoflurane can artificially depress hematologic values, particularly packed cell volume (PCV) and red blood cell (RBC) and white blood cell (WBC) numbers.[33] Isoflurane should be administered using an open anesthetic system at a flow rate of 1.5 to 2 L of oxygen/min and a 5% minimal alveolar concentration (MAC) until the animal is relaxed. The patient is usually anesthetized in 1 to 3 minutes. Patients can be maintained under anesthesia at 1.5 to 3% MAC. Dose-dependent cardiopulmonary depression is an uncommon side effect of isoflurane use.[51]

Other inhalant anesthetics can also be used for the ferret. Methoxyflurane and halothane have both been used in a similar manner as isoflurane.[52] However, both have caused serious side effects.[51] Methoxyflurane is a potential nephrotoxin and is associated with prolonged induction and recovery.[51] Halothane use can lead to dose-dependent cardiopulmonary depression and myocardial sensitization and has a potential for hepatotoxicity.[51] The safest inhalant anesthetic for both the patient and anesthetist is isoflurane. Inhalation equipment must be maintained properly and adequate ventilation provided to prevent human exposure.

Injectable anesthetics can be used in the ferret. See Table 5-1 for common drug combinations and dosages. The most frequently used injectable anesthetic is ketamine, either alone or in combination with other drugs. Ketamine use can lead to hypersalivation, and premedication with atropine or glycopyrrolate is recommended.[50] Ketamine combinations usually provide a 30- to 90-minute surgical plane of anesthesia. Ketamine can cause delayed recovery from anesthesia and has also been associated with seizures in susceptible animals in the author's experience (Purcell); however, healthy ferrets tolerate this drug well. Acepromazine or acepromazine-butorphanol can be used in combination with ketamine to provide more muscle relaxation.[53] Exercise caution when using acepromazine, because its vasodilative effects can result in increased body heat loss.[54] Acepromazine given at the high end of its dosage range can lead to prolonged recovery time.[11]

Medetomidine (Domitor, Orion Corporation, Espoo, Finland) is a relatively new injectable anesthetic. It is fully reversible with atipamezole (Antisedan, Orion Corporation, Espoo, Finland).[34] It can be used alone for short procedures, such as blood collection, or in various combinations with ketamine and butorphanol for longer procedures or those requiring analgesia, such as minor surgical procedures. Apnea with resultant hypoxia has occasionally been seen with medetomidine use.[34]

Tiletamine is another relatively new anesthetic agent. It is usually used in combination with zolazepam, xylazine, and/or butorphanol. Side effects with these combinations include decreased pulse rate, cardiac arrhythmias (e.g., respiratory sinus arrhythmia and second-degree atrioventricular heart block), and depression of respiratory function.[55] To counteract hypersalivation with the tiletamine–zolazepam combination, pretreat with atropine or glycopyrrolate.[50] Because of the potentially serious side effects, tiletamine is not considered by the authors to be a safe anesthetic choice.

Diazepam is used primarily for seizure control, but it can also be used in combination with ketamine or butorphanol for sedation. Diazepam can cause excitation, pacing, restlessness, anxiety, and sensitivity to noise when used alone at a dose of 3 mg/kg body weight.[53,56]

Xylazine works as a sedative or tranquilizer for short procedures in the ferret.[53] Its sedative and analgesic properties are increased if it is combined with butorphanol.[56] In combination with ketamine, it has proved fatal on occasion even for apparently healthy animals.[11] It is not recommended for use in the ferret for this reason.

Barbiturates have long been used in laboratory animal research. However, because of unpredictability in regard to reactions with other drugs, as well as multisystemic depressive effects, their use should be avoided in ferrets.[10,51]

Routes of Administration

Injectable anesthetics can be given intramuscularly (IM) or intravenously (IV), at the clinician's discretion. Because of the small amount of muscle mass, the volume of IM medications should be kept small.

Inhalant anesthesia can be administered by mask using a nonrebreathing anesthetic system.[51] An induction tank is useful for the active, less cooperative ferret. Patients can be maintained with a mask for the duration of the anesthesia or be intubated.[11] Oxygen should be maintained at 1.5 to 2 L/min. It is generally not necessary to use any preanesthetic agents before the use of inhalants. Complete recovery time is dependent on the condition of the pet and the length of the procedure, but in healthy animals it has been observed to be approximately 5 to 10 minutes.[11,24]

Endotracheal Intubation

Ferrets should be adequately anesthetized before intubation is attempted. Lidocaine (0.05 ml) can be applied to the larynx to prevent laryngospasm.[11] Lidocaine-based sprays should be avoided to prevent aspiration. A cotton swab is dampened with lidocaine for application to the larynx and a laryngoscope used to visualize the larynx. A headlamp leaves the hands free while providing illumination of the area.[51] A 2- to 3-mm uncuffed endotracheal (ET) tube is used in female ferrets and a 3- to 3.5-mm uncuffed tube in males.[11,50] A silicon-cuffed tube (Aire-Cuf, Bivona, Gary, IN) is available that can be used in ferrets.[24] Placement of the ET tube is similar to the procedure for cats: place the patient in ventral recumbency and extend the neck, holding the mouth open with the head tilted upward. It is helpful to have an assistant hold the mouth open with gauze strips.[18] Assess correct placement by direct observation of the tube passing into the glottis, condensation within a clear tube or on a piece of cold metal held before the opening, or air movement seen from the end of the tube.[51]

Avoid multiple attempts at intubation, as this can lead to laryngeal swelling and hemorrhage.[51] When the tube is in place, tie a gauze strip to the tube just caudal to the canine teeth and fasten around the nose or behind the ears of the patient.

Depth of Anesthesia

Anesthesia depth in ferrets is measured as it is in cats and dogs. Loss of the palpebral and corneal reflexes and jaw tone is most commonly used.[51] Test analgesia via the pinch reflex on the toe webs. Slow and regular respiration and a mildly decreased but regular heart rate and blood pressure are normal for a moderate depth of anesthesia. An esophageal stethoscope or respiratory monitors within the anesthetic tubing enhance detection of problems. Pulse rate can be monitored with a pulse oximeter clipped to the tail.[48] Cardiac output can be tracked audibly with a Doppler ultrasound blood pressure monitor (Parks Medical Electronics, Aloha, OR).[50] Electrocardiographic monitoring is also an option, although the alligator clips should be modified with flattened teeth for the patient's comfort.[31]

Anesthetic Overdose

In general, ferrets are resilient anesthetic subjects, and with routine monitoring, anesthetic overdose is a rare occurrence. Signs of overdose include flaccid jaw tone, lack of corneal reflex, and increasing depression of the cardiac, pulmonary, and central nervous systems. If the patient is exhibiting these signs, cease all anesthesia immediately and administer reversal agents if appropriate. Treat the ferret according to the animal's requirements—for example, respiratory support for hypoxia and pulmonary depression, fluid therapy for a decrease in blood pressure, lidocaine and epinephrine for cardiac arrest. Heat lamps and warm-water–circulating pads or an incubator are essential to keep body temperature regulated. Monitor the patient carefully to avoid hyperthermia caused by overzealous warming. Cardiopulmonary resuscitation (CPR) is appropriate in the event of cardiac arrest.

Analgesia

Uncontrolled pain leads to increased glucocorticoid release and generalized stress on all systems of the body. In the presence of pain, ferrets
exhibit depression, squinting, crying, lameness, anorexia, inability to
curl into a normal sleep position, aggression, and decreased activity.[12]
Proper pain management is essential for the success of medical and
surgical interventions.

Patients provided with preemptive pain relief, preferably preoperatively or interoperatively, exhibit better appetite and a quicker return to
normal behavior upon recovery.[50] For pre- and postsurgical pain management, opioid agonist–antagonist drugs, such as buprenorphine or
butorphanol, are used. Naloxone is the appropriate reversal agent for
these medications. Nonsteroidal anti-inflammatory drugs (NSAIDs)
such as aspirin, flunixin meglumine, or carprofen are useful for dental
or orthopedic pain. Avoid using NSAIDs concurrently with corticosteroids or in the presence of gastric disorders.[12]

Table 5-1
Anesthetic and Analgesic Agents

Drugs and dosages listed are those most commonly used in ferrets. Dosages, applications, and duration of use may vary from case to case. Some dosages are based on empirical use and not pharmacological studies.

DRUG DOSE/ROUTE	COMMENTS
Acepromazine[2,3,*]	
0.1–0.25 mg/kg SC, IM	Preanesthetic; light sedation.
0.2–0.5 mg/kg SC, IM	Tranquilization; the lower end of this dose may be used with 25–35 mg/kg of ketamine for short-term anesthesia.
Aspirin[3,*]	
0.5–20 mg/kg q 8–24h PO	
Atipamezole[5,*]	
0.4 mg/kg IM	Reversal agent for medetomidine. This dose is used to reverse 0.08 mg/kg medetomidine. Normal calculation is same *volume* (not mg dose) of atipamezole used as volume of medetomidine used.
Atropine sulfate[3,4,6,*]	
0.04–0.05 mg/kg SC, IM, IV	Preanesthetic.
Buprenorphine[1,2,*]	
0.01–0.03 mg/kg q 8–12h SC, IM, IV	Analgesic.
Butorphanol tartrate[1,2,5*]	
0.05–0.5 mg/kg q 8–12h SC, IM	Analgesic; can be used pre-, intra-, or postoperatively.

NOTE: IM = intramuscularly; IV = intravenously; IT = intratracheally; PO = per os, orally; SC = subcutaneously

Brown, S.A. Personal experience using this agent in practice situations. These listings are accompanied by pertinent comments based on anecdotal experiences.

continued

0.1 mg/kg SC, IM

Use at this dose in combination with ketamine (5 mg/kg IM) and medetomidine (0.08 mg/kg IM) for anesthesia with analgesia.

Carprofen*
1 mg/kg *q* 12–24h PO

Nonsteroidal antiinflammatory drug (NSAID) with fewer gastrointestinal effects than flunixin. Use with caution in ferrets with enteritis or gastritis. Do not use in conjunction with corticosteroids.

Diazepam[1,2,3,4,*]
1–2 mg/kg PO, SC, IM, IV, as needed

For seizure control and sedation.

1.0–1.5 mg/kg/h continuous IV

For control of status epilepticus.

Fentanyl/droperidol[4,7]
0.15 ml/kg IM

For minor surgical procedures and deep sedation.

Flunixin meglumine[1,6,*]
0.5–2.0 mg/kg *q* 12–24h PO, IM, IV

NSAID. Use with caution in ferrets with enteritis or gastritis. Do not use in conjunction with corticosteroids. Be cautious using it for more than 5 days continuously as possibility of gastrointestinal ulcers exists. Injectable form can be administered orally in a palatable syrup.

Glycopyrrolate[6]
0.01 mg/kg IM

Preanesthetic.

Ketamine[2,3,4,6,7,*]

May require premedication with atropine due to hypersalivation.

10–20 mg/kg IM

Tranquilization.

25–40 mg/kg IM

Anesthetic dose; however, best if used in combination with an analgesic.

Ketamine + acepromazine[2,3,*]
20–40 mg/kg ketamine IM
+ 0.2–0.35 mg/kg acepromazine SC, IM

Anesthesia.

Ketamine + diazepam[2,3,4,*]
25–35 mg/kg ketamine IM +   Anesthesia.
  2–3 mg/kg diazepam IM

Ketoprofen[*]
1 mg/kg q 24h PO, IM   NSAID. Same cautions as listed for flunixin meglumine.

Medetomidine[5,*]
0.08 mg/kg IM   Sedative for noninvasive procedures. Reverse with
    atipamezole at 0.40 mg/kg IM.

Medetomidine + ketamine + butorphanol[5,*]
0.08 mg/kg medetomidine IM   Anesthesia for short surgical procedures.
  + 5 mg/kg ketamine IM +   All three drugs are given at the same time
  0.10 mg/kg butorphanol IM   and may be combined in the same syringe.
    Reverse with atipamezole at 0.40 mg/kg IM.

Meperidine[1,6]
5–20 mg/kg q 2–4h SC, IM, IV   Analgesic.

Morphine[6]
0.5–5.0 mg/kg q 2–6h SC, IM   Analgesic.

Nalbuphine[6]
0.5–1.5 mg/kg q 2–3h IM, IV   Analgesic.

Oxymorphone[1,6]
0.05–0.20 mg/kg q 8–12h SC,   Analgesic.
  IM, IV

Pentazocine[1,6]
5–10 mg/kg q 4h IM   Analgesic.

Phenobarbitol elixir[1,*]
1–2 mg/kg q 8–12h PO   For seizure control. Titrate dose for maintenance.

Tiletamine-zolazepam[6,8]
12–22 mg/kg IM   Sedation at lower dose; use higher dose for minor
    surgical procedures.

continued

References

1. Smith, D.A., and Burgman, P.M. Formulary. In Hillyer, E.V., and Quesenberry, K.E., eds., Ferrets, rabbits and rodents: Clinical medicine and surgery, pp. 394–397. Philadelphia: W.B. Saunders; 1997.

2. Carpenter, J.W., Mashima, T.Y., and Rupiper, D.J. Exotic animal formulary. Manhattan, KS: Greystone; 1996.

3. Johnson-Delaney, C.A. Exotic companion medicine handbood. Lake Worth, FL: Wingers Publishing.

4. Hawk, D.F., and Leary, S.L. Formulary for laboratory animals. Ames: Iowa State Press; 1995.

5. Ko, J.C.H., Heaton-Jones, T.G., and Nicklin, C.F. Evaluation of the sedative and cardiorespiratory effects of medetomidine, medetomidine-butorphanol, medetomidine-ketamine and medetomidine-butorphanol-ketamine in ferrets. JAAHA 33:438–448; 1997.

6. Heard, D.J. Principles and techniques of anesthesia and analgesia for exotic practice. Vet Clin North Am/Small Anim Pract 23:1301–1327; 1993.

7. Flecknell, P.A. Laboratory animal anesthesia. London: Academic Press; 1987.

8. Payton, A.J., and Pick, J.R. Evaluation of a combination of tiletamine and zolazepam as an anesthetic for ferrets. Lab Anim Sci 39:243–246; 1989.

6

Surgery

Introduction

As ferrets become more popular, the number of surgical procedures necessary for their continued health grows. Many of the surgical procedures used in dogs and cats are performed in the ferret with consideration for their smaller size and peculiarities of anatomy. In all procedures, standard aseptic preparation should be followed to prevent postoperative infection.

Presurgical blood work is recommended before any procedure. In ferrets younger than 3 years, a minimum baseline includes a complete blood cell (CBC) count, blood glucose, and hepatic enzyme levels. Ferrets older than 3 years should ideally have a CBC count, chemistry panel, and whole-body radiographs preoperatively. In the event that cardiac abnormalities are noted, perform echocardiography and a complete cardiac workup before anesthesia.[54]

Ferrets have a short intestinal tract, which empties rapidly. To avoid the possibility of vomiting and aspiration, a 4- to 6-hour fast is recommended before anesthesia.[49] A longer fast can result in hypoglycemia in older patients.

Place intravenous (IV) or intraosseous (IO) catheters preoperatively. An open IV line is essential in the event of emergency. Perioperative fluids should be warmed prior to and during administration. The maintenance fluid rate in the ferret is estimated as 70 ml/kg/day.[12] Syringe pumps or flow meters are recommended for accurate fluid administration. Either lactated Ringer's solution (LRS) or isotonic saline is appropriate. Older ferrets (older than 3 years) may benefit from 2.5 to 5% dextrose in saline solution perioperatively if preoperative blood glucose levels are not within normal limits. Monitor fluid rates carefully to prevent pulmonary edema.

Ferrets are particularly susceptible to hypothermia because of their small body size. Monitor body temperature with a digital rectal thermometer throughout anesthesia and maintain with warm-water–circulating heating pads set to 102 to 104°F, hot water bottles, and/or warmed towels.[57] Avoid electric heating pads, as they can lead to burns.[51] Keep preparation and surgical time to a minimum. Warm any fluids used within the abdominal cavity. Modify routine aseptic surgical preparation to decrease the risk of hypothermia. Shave the hair carefully to avoid lacerating the skin. Expose only the amount of skin necessary for the procedure to decrease heat loss. Hair regrowth can take up to 3 months in the ferret. Use small amounts of water to scrub, and avoid or minimize the use of alcohol.

Express the bladder to prevent urine contamination during surgery. Apply artificial tears ointment to the corneas to prevent drying and ulceration. Administer analgesics preoperatively for optimal pain management.

The patient's cardiopulmonary activity should be monitored with any combination of the following: stethoscope and/or esophageal stethoscope, pulse oximeter, or Doppler ultrasound blood pressure monitor (Parks Medical Electronics, Aloha, OR).[34,50] Electrocardiographic monitoring is also an option, but the alligator clips should be modified with flattened teeth for the comfort of the patient.[31] Emergency drugs (epinephrine, lidocaine) should be drawn up preoperatively in case of emergency. Dilution is usually necessary because of the small volumes required. Insulin syringes are accurate to a volume of 0.01 cc and are useful in this regard.[57]

The ferret should be kept in a quiet, warm, well-ventilated enclosure during recovery. A small-animal or pediatric incubator set at 78°F (25.6°C) works well.[58] Continue to monitor body temperature. Provide a towel or small blanket for hiding to increase the animal's comfort. After routine surgical procedures, provide water as soon as the patient is conscious. Offer food 2 hours postoperatively unless gastrointestinal

(GI) surgery has been performed. Feeding recommendations in the event of digestive tract surgery are mentioned with the individual procedure. In the event that the patient has not eaten within 4 hours of recovery, assist-feed a high-protein liquid diet to prevent hypoglycemia.

Instruments and Supplies

Given the small area exposed for surgery, strong environmental lighting such as with halogen examination or surgery lights is recommended for good visualization of the tissues. Magnification, especially with an attached light source, is also recommended for surgery on these small patients. Binocular loupes are available through hobby shops. A modified hobby loupe with an attached light source and interchangeable lenses is available (MDS, Inc., Brandon, FL), as well as one designed for surgeons (SurgiTelR, General Scientific Corp., Ann Arbor, MI).[57]

A minimum recommended set of surgical instruments for ferrets includes mosquito forceps, small Carmalt clamps, fine-tipped needle holders, small Metzenbaum scissors, ophthalmic scissors of varying types, ophthalmic forceps, No. 15 blades, and abdominal retractors (Heiss blunt retractors or Alm).[18] Microsurgical instruments are ideal for high-quality ferret surgery. Examples include long jeweler's forceps No. 3, round-handled microsurgical forceps, Castroviejo pen needle holder 5.25 inch, and Tew Barraquer scissors curved 7 inch.

Sterile cotton-tipped applicators can be used for blunt dissection. Small sterile gauze pads allow more precise monitoring of blood loss. Control hemorrhage with Gelfoam (The Upjohn Co., Kalamazoo, MI) or Surgicel (Johnson & Johnson Healthcare Systems, Piscataway, NJ). Hemostatic clips for hemostasis are useful and timesaving.

Swedged-on synthetic suture material from 4–0 to 8–0 should be available on both taper and cutting needles. Catgut is not recommended because of a tendency to induce granuloma formation and dehiscence.[18] Absorbable monofilament or braided synthetic may be used internally, at the surgeon's discretion. Use tissue glue to reinforce subcuticular closure. Close skin with staples or 4–0 nonabsorbable suture or use a subcuticular layer with no skin closure.

General Considerations

Ferret skin is thick and tough, requiring slightly more pressure for incisions than dog or cat skin. Tent the abdominal wall before making a stab incision to avoid the spleen, which is often enlarged in this species. Significant hemorrhage can occur if the incision is made off the midline. Ferrets cannot sustain large amounts of blood loss. Hemostasis is critical.[18]

Electrosurgery is useful in the ferret. High-frequency electric current provides either a cutting blade or coagulation with minimal tissue damage. The use of electrosurgery decreases surgery time and provides rapid hemostasis. Overuse should be avoided to prevent heat buildup in the tissues.[57]

Abdominal diseases, including a variety of neoplasms, bladder disease, gastric foreign bodies, and hepatic disorders, are common in ferrets. For this reason, it is important to examine the entire abdominal contents whenever abdominal surgery is performed. In particular, examine the adrenal glands, pancreas, ovaries, uterus, bladder, stomach, spleen, mesenteric lymph nodes, and liver. If care is taken to keep exposed tissues moistened and covered, it is possible to exteriorize much of the abdominal viscera for examination without ill effect to the patient. Biopsy specimens of all suspicious-looking tissues should be taken.

Adrenalectomy

Indications

Adrenal-associated endocrinopathy is one of the most common disorders in ferrets.[59,60] Surgical removal is the treatment of choice in otherwise healthy animals. See chapter 7, Endocrine System—Adrenal Glands, for the surgical qualifications.

Anatomy

The left adrenal is found within the sublumbar fat just cranial and medial to the anterior pole of the left kidney. The phrenicoabdominal vein crosses the gland. The ventral surface can be visualized in most ferrets. The right adrenal is located by lifting the caudal pole of the caudate lobe of the liver overlying the anterior pole of the right kidney. After gently lifting this liver lobe, the adrenal is found on the midline attached directly to the right dorsal aspect of the vena cava. Both glands are normally light pink in color, homogeneous in appearance, and approximately 2 to 4 mm wide and 4 to 6 mm long (figure 15).[42]

Procedure

Place an IV or IO catheter with a slow drip of lactated Ringer's solution (25 ml/kg/hr) 30 minutes before surgery. Administer preoperative analgesics (see chapter 5, Analgesia). Place the patient in dorsal recumbency and aseptically prepare the ventrum from xiphoid to pubis. Make a ventral midline incision from just caudal to the xiphoid to the pubis.

Examine both adrenal glands thoroughly for abnormalities. Note that the abnormal gland is often not grossly enlarged; changes can be subtle. The appearance of lumps, discoloration, cysts, or gross enlargement is cause for removal (figure 15). If both glands are involved, remove the left adrenal gland completely and perform a subtotal or complete removal of the right adrenal gland, as appropriate for the situation.[42,49]

The left adrenal is easily located and visualized by blunt dissection. Ligate the phrenicoabdominal vein on either side of the gland before removal. Hemostasis with gentle pressure or Gelfoam (The Upjohn

Co., Kalamazoo, MI) is usually sufficient to control bleeding from small blood vessels. Hemostatic clips are useful for hemostasis in well-vascularized tumors. When all the vessels have been ligated, the gland is removed by blunt dissection with cotton-tipped applicators, which minimize trauma to the surrounding tissues.[42]

Locate the right adrenal gland under the caudal pole of the caudate lobe of the liver. Sharp incision of the thin hepatorenal ligament allows better access to the gland.[42] It is difficult to remove the right adrenal gland because of its close association with the vena cava, but with careful dissection a large portion if not all of the gland can be excised. Sterile cotton-tipped applicators are an excellent tool for blunt dissection of the surrounding tissues. Be prepared for vascular surgery when removing the right adrenal. When the gland has been isolated by blunt dissection, leaving only the attachment to the vena cava, apply a neonatal Satinsky vena cava clamp.[42] Identify the plane of dissection between the adrenal gland and the vessel. Gently dissect the gland free. Before removing the clamp, make a "taco" of Gelfoam (Upjohn, Kalamazoo, MI) wrapped in Surgicel (Johnson & Johnson Healthcare Systems, Piscataway, NJ).[42] Remove the clamp, placing the "taco" over the vena cava and applying gentle pressure for 5 minutes to provide hemostasis.[42] If an incision is inadvertently made in the wall of the vena cava during dissection, close with 8–0 to 10–0 monofilament suture on an atraumatic needle in a simple continuous pattern and then apply the "taco."[42] Leave the "taco" in place during abdominal closure.

Alternatively, hemostatic clips can be placed between the right adrenal gland and the vena cava when the gland has been freed from the surrounding tissues.[42] The adrenal gland is transected along the clip. This technique does not provide complete removal of the glandular tissue.

In the rare event that the right adrenal gland has compromised the vessel lumen and collateral circulation is already in place, vena caval ligation can be performed.[49,61] This procedure should be performed only if no other option is available. Discuss this option with the owner preoperatively, as the incidence of fatalities after this procedure is high. Triple ligate the vena cava cranial to the renal vessels and just cranial to the right adrenal gland. Transect carefully, leaving the double ligation on the remaining vascular stumps. Congestion of the right kidney may be noted. Localized metastasis to the caudate liver lobe may require a liver lobectomy as well.[61] Histopathology is highly recommended, as liver metastasis is more commonly caused by insulinoma.

In male ferrets with urethral obstruction, examine the neck of the bladder for paraurethral cysts and enlargement of prostatic tissue (figure 17). Obtain biopsy specimens of any abnormal tissue. Drain cysts and remove or reduce if possible. Perform cytology and culture the fluid. Marsupializing the cysts to the bladder or abdominal wall to allow postoperative drainage is seldom necessary but can be a treatment option.[62] The prognosis is poor in ferrets with severe cystic paraurethral tissue.[63]

If the adrenal gland(s) is inoperable because of location or size, obtain a biopsy specimen to determine whether postsurgical chemotherapy is warranted (see chapter 7, Endocrine System). Some adrenal tumors develop blood-filled sinuses because of invasion of the vena cava. Exsanguination is a serious risk with biopsy in these cases.[18]

Close the abdomen with 4–0 absorbable synthetic monofilament suture material in the muscle layer and monofilament nylon or skin staples in the skin. Remove skin sutures in 7 to 10 days. Alternatively, the subcutaneous and subcuticular tissues are closed with 4–0 or 5–0 absorbable monofilament in a continuous pattern and skin sutures are unnecessary. Treat postoperatively with a single dose of dexamethasone (1 mg/kg). Continue corticosteroid therapy 24 hours after operation with oral prednisone (0.1 mg/kg) every 24 hours for 3 days, then every other day for three doses. Postsurgical analgesics are also recommended.

Postsurgical considerations

Complications of this surgery include postoperative lethargy, anorexia, and death. Lethargy and anorexia should be investigated for underlying causes, including hypoglycemia, postoperative pain, blood loss, and decreased blood cortisol levels. Iatrogenic Addison's disease is a distinct possibility in bilateral adrenal gland removal. Cortisol levels should be monitored routinely immediately after operation and 5 to 7 days after surgery. Postoperative fatalities have been attributed to subclinical cardiomyopathy, insufficient cortisol related to iatrogenic Addison's disease, thromboembolic disease caused by manipulation of the vena cava, disseminated intravascular coagulation (DIC), complete obstruction of the vena cava without sufficient collateral circulation, exsanguination related to surgery, hypoglycemia, persistent aplastic anemia, and metastatic invasion of the abdomen.[18,49]

In the uneventful recovery, the patient can return to a normal diet in 2 hours. If the ferret is not eating on its own, use strained-meat baby food, a/d (Hill's Pet Products, Topeka, KS), or feline critical care products fed by syringe every 2 to 4 hours. Maintenance fluid therapy should be continued until the patient is eating on its own. The patient is discharged when normal eating and elimination habits have resumed, usually 1 to 2 days postsurgically. If the entire or a sufficient amount of the tumor was removed, the swollen vulva will return to normal within 2 weeks, and hair growth will resume in 1 to 4 months.[42]

If vena caval ligation was performed, the patient should be monitored carefully for signs of kidney failure. Hind limb weakness and hematuria are common sequelae but should resolve in 2 to 3 days.

Anal Sacculectomy

Indications

This procedure is popularly known as "descenting." In the United States, it is usually performed in ferrets 4 to 6 weeks of age at the breeding farms before sale to the public.[54] Removal of the anal glands is an unnecessary elective procedure in ferrets and in fact does little to remove body odor (see chapter 2). However, if an adult ferret expresses these glands frequently or develops an infection, bilateral removal will resolve the situation. Anal gland resection may also be necessary in the event of neoplasia. Squamous cell carcinoma has been reported affecting the anus.[59] In cases of infection, preoperative antibiotics for 7 to 10 days decrease the size of the affected gland(s).[18] Anal sacculectomy can be performed at neutering or as needed in the older ferret.

Anatomy

The paired anal glands are located at 4 and 8 o'clock on either side of the anus. Magnification may help visualize the small openings in the mucocutaneous junction.

Procedure

When the anal gland openings are visualized, the duct and surrounding skin and mucocutaneous tissue are grasped with a mosquito forceps. With a No. 15 blade, a shallow incision is made around the forceps tip. With the tip of the scalpel or a sterile cotton-tipped applicator, the tissue overlying the glands is gently scraped away. The first 3 to 5 mm of perianal tissue is quite tough, but the fascial plane surrounding the gland is easily dissected.[64] Once the gland is exposed, it can be bluntly dissected from the perianal tissues and anal sphincter. Try to remove the anal sac intact to avoid contaminating the surgical environment with the overwhelming odor. If the gland ruptures, flush the area with sterile saline.[64] When the glands have been removed, the incision is left open to heal.

In the majority of cases, recovery from this procedure is unremarkable. When anal glands are not completely removed or are scarred by chronic infections, draining tracts can occur in the perianal tissues.[64] Carefully explore the draining tract. The sac wall can be identified by the mucosal appearance. Remove all abnormal tissue by resection or blunt dissection, taking care to avoid the anal sphincter.[64] All secretory tissue must be removed or the draining tract will recur.

Postsurgical considerations

If surgery is performed properly, with care to remain in the appropriate fascial plane, there are few adverse consequences. Persistent postoperative hemorrhage can occur but ceases spontaneously with gentle pressure.[54] Rectal prolapse and fecal incontinence happen rarely unless trauma to the sphincter muscles is excessive.[54] Malformed stools and fistulous tracts result from incompletely removed glands, regardless of the patient's age at the time of surgery.[64]

Cesarean Section

Indications

Dystocia caused by uterine inertia, protracted labor, an oversized fetus, or retained placenta requires a cesarean section to preserve the lives of both the offspring and the jill.[5] Jills carrying more than 13 kits or receiving inadequate nutrition in the last 10 days of pregnancy may develop pregnancy toxemia.[20] An immediate cesarean section is necessary if illness is noted at day 39 to 41 of pregnancy (see chapter 7, Urogenital System).[20] Struvite urolithiasis is also an indication for surgery, because straining can lead to vaginal prolapse (see chapter 7, Urogenital System).[20] If cystotomy is indicated within 24 hours of the due date, a cesarean can be done simultaneously.[20] Both conditions require fluid therapy during surgery. Normal gestation in ferrets is 41 to 42 days; any longer gestation may require surgical intervention to save the kits and perhaps the jill if medical induction of labor is unsuccessful (see chapter 7, Urogenital System).[5]

The prognosis for surgical recovery and possible sequelae should be discussed with the owner in advance. Simultaneous ovariohysterectomy may be in the best interest of the jill, especially if the fetuses have died or infection is present.

Anatomy

The ferret has a bicornate uterus, with a short body fused just cranial to the cervix.[7] In pregnancy, the horns can extend cranially to the rib cage.

Procedure

Place an IV or IO catheter and administer LRS or saline preoperatively at 25 ml/kg/h. If it will not place undue stress on the jill, place the ferret in dorsal recumbency and clip the abdomen from xiphoid to pubis before anesthesia, to minimize fetal exposure to the anesthetic. The best anesthetic for this procedure is isoflurane without any preanesthetic. When the jill has been anesthetized, aseptically prepare the ventral abdomen. Make a ventral midline incision just caudal to the umbilicus to the pubis. Gently reflect the enlarged mammary tissue to avoid damage. The uterus may be pressing against the abdominal wall, so take care to tent the linea alba before entering the abdomen. Exteriorize the horns separately. Remove kits via an incision midway down each horn, milking the kits to the opening. As each fetus is removed, the umbilicus is clamped and severed 2 to 3 mm from the kit's abdominal wall. Open the amniotic sac to allow the kit to begin breathing, and hand off to an assistant for resuscitation as needed. Remove each placenta after each fetus, using gentle traction. Before closure, palpate the entire uterus to be certain that all fetuses and placentas have been removed. The uterus will already be contracting at this point. Close the uterine incisions with 4–0 to 6–0 synthetic absorbable suture on a taper needle. Appose the edges with an inverting continuous Cushing pattern followed by a continuous Lembert oversew. Before returning the uterus to the abdomen, inspect the incision and flush with warmed sterile saline. If the uterus is flaccid, with no evidence of contracting, administer oxytocin (0.2–3 USP units/kg subcutaneous [SC] or intramuscular [IM]). Close the abdominal wall with 4–0 synthetic absorbable suture. Place a final layer of sutures in the subcuticular tissues with 4–0 or 5–0 absorbable suture to prevent the kits from having a chance to disturb external sutures. Alternatively, place staples in the skin, which will not be disturbed by the kits.

In the event that an ovariohysterectomy is necessary, the procedure is followed through exteriorization of the uterine horns. Break down the suspensory and broad ligaments, leaving the blood vessels intact while freeing all other attachments. Palpate the cervix for the presence of a kit. If one is present, gently manipulate it until it is back in the uterine body. Place two hemostatic clamps across each ovarian pedicle and three clamps across the body of the uterus just cranial to the cervix. Divide the uterine body and the pedicles between the clamps, and hand the reproductive tract to assistants for removal and resuscitation of the fetuses. At this point, the ovarian pedicles and uterine stump are ligated. Complete the abdominal closure as described above.

Open the gravid uterine horns with a scalpel or scissors, taking care not to lacerate the fetuses. Remove the amniotic sac, suture the umbilicus on each neonate, and resuscitate as needed.

When the kits have been delivered, administer interoperative analgesics to the jill.

Postoperative considerations

If there is evidence of a uterine infection at the time of surgery, there is a possibility for peritonitis to develop. Perform a bacterial culture and sensitivity on the wall of the uterus. Appropriate antibiotic therapy should be started immediately. Observe for postoperative signs of stump pyometra as well, which includes depression, lethargy, foul-smelling vaginal discharge, swollen vulva, palpable uterine stump within abdomen, anorexia, and fever (see chapter 7, Urogenital System).[19,64] Toxemic or debilitated jills require intensive care, including assisted feeding of a high-fat, high-protein diet and maintenance of hydration and body temperature.[20] The first 24 hours are critical to the jill's survival.[20] If the jill's milk does not come in and no foster mother is available, or if the kits are younger than 40 days of gestation, euthanasia of the kits is the most humane option, because hand rearing is seldom successful.[20] Toxemic jills do not produce milk.

Cystotomy

Indications

Ferrets can develop urolithiasis, most commonly struvite.[65] The presence of calculi requires surgical removal (see chapter 7, Urogenital System). Diverticula present in the dorsal apex of the bladder require surgical removal if clinical signs of disease exist (figure 16) (see chapter 7, Urogenital System). Bladder rupture is rare but may occur with trauma to the tissues or unrelieved obstruction. Fluid therapy to correct electrolyte imbalances will stabilize the patient until corrective surgery can be performed.

Anatomy

The bladder is adjacent to the abdominal wall just cranial to the pelvic inlet. Dorsally it is adjacent to the caudal small intestine, the descending colon, and the uterine horns in the female. It is fixed to the abdominal wall with three ligaments, lateral right and left and the middle ligament of the bladder.[7]

Procedure

Place an IV or IO catheter and administer warmed saline at 25 ml/kg/hr. Administer preoperative analgesics (see chapter 5). Aseptically prepare the ventral abdomen with the anesthetized ferret in dorsal recumbency. Make a caudal midline incision in the female, a parapreputial incision in the male, taking care not to incise the bladder.[66] Isolate the bladder from the abdominal contents with laparotomy pads or sterile gauze.[66] Place retention sutures in the cranial end of the bladder and reflect caudally to expose the dorsal surface.[66] Examine the apex of the bladder for diverticula.[19] Empty the bladder via cystocentesis, then make a 2- to 3-cm incision in an avascular portion of the ventral bladder wall.[66] A spoon or forceps can be used to remove

urethral calculi.[66] Use retropulsion via a catheter placed into the urethral opening to flush sand and calculi from the neck of the bladder
and the urethra.[66] Obtain cultures of the bladder wall and calculi and
biopsy specimens of any abnormal tissue. Flush the bladder with warm
sterile saline solution before closure.[66] Use 4–0 synthetic absorbable
monofilament suture on an atraumatic needle for double-layer closure,
using a simple continuous suture pattern, followed by an inverting pattern.[42] Flush the abdomen with sterile saline and close routinely.
Submit calculi for analysis.

If a cystic diverticulum is present in the bladder wall, the same
approach is used to resect the structures, making every attempt to
retain functional structure of the bladder[67] (figure 17). Submit the
resected tissues for histopathology.

Postoperative considerations

Postoperative care includes 24 to 48 hours of IV fluid diuresis and
analgesia provided as needed.[42] Administer antibiotics according to
culture and sensitivity results for a minimum of 14 days. Convert the
patient to a diet that has high-quality meat protein and very little plant
protein.[68] Urinary acidifiers are not necessary.

Cystopexy and Cystotomy Tube Placement

Indications

Cystopexy and cystotomy tube placement is used to bypass the urethra
temporarily or to permanently resolve urethral obstruction from
urolithiasis or paraurethral cysts at the neck of the bladder.

Anatomy: See Cystotomy

Procedure

Administer warmed LRS or saline solution at 25 ml/kg/hr. Preoperative analgesia is recommended (see chapter 5, Anesthesia). Aseptically

prepare the ventral abdomen with the anesthetized ferret in dorsal recumbency. Make a ventral midline incision from xiphoid to pubis. Perform a complete abdominal exploratory examination before approaching the bladder. In particular, examine both adrenal glands closely, because adrenal gland endocrinopathy is often associated with paraurethral and prostatic cysts. Remove or obtain biopsy specimens of abnormal tissues as needed. If cystic structures are present, remove the contents interoperatively.[42] Obtain a biopsy of the prostatic tissue if enlarged.[69] Preplace two sutures of 4–0 absorbable suture attaching the bladder muscularis and serosal layers, avoiding the mucosa, to the internal and external abdominal oblique muscles.[70] The needle passes through the bladder layers, exiting 5 to 8 mm from the entry point, then enters the adjoining abdominal musculature, again exiting 5 to 8 mm from the entry point.[70] Place the second suture parallel to the first.[70] Do NOT tie the sutures at this point, but rather leave long suture ends. Use a No. 15 blade to make a stab incision through the body wall and skin at the center of the four preplaced sutures.[70] Insert a 3.5 to 5 French soft red rubber or a clear feeding tube from the skin into the abdomen. Make a stab incision into the empty bladder at the center of the preplaced sutures.[70] Insert 2 to 3 cm of the tip of the tube into the bladder lumen.[70] Tighten and tie the preplaced sutures, with care to avoid pressure necrosis.[70] Secure the catheter to the skin with a nonabsorbable "Chinese finger trap" suture pattern.[70] Cut the tube 2 cm from the skin.[70] Place two nonabsorbable stay sutures at the anchor point of the Chinese finger trap on opposite points of the catheter's exit point to prevent migration of the tube.[70] These sutures remain until the catheter is removed (usually 1 to 3 months).[70]

Postsurgical considerations

Keep the patient in the hospital 5 to 7 days for observation.[70] Flush the catheter frequently with a syringe of sterile saline to remove blood, cells, and protein debris.[70] Administer analgesics such as butorphanol as needed postsurgically for pain management (see chapter 5). Continue IV or IO fluid therapy until electrolyte imbalances are corrected.

Continue antibiotics as needed, based on culture and sensitivity results. Nutritional support may be necessary as well. Prevent urine scald by frequent application of petroleum jelly around the catheter.[70]

When the ferret regains the ability to urinate via the urethra, remove the cystotomy tube. With the ferret under general anesthesia, aseptically prepare the area around the tube from the umbilicus to the pubis. Perform a ventral midline incision, remove the catheter, and break down the bladder or abdominal wall adhesions via sharp dissection.[70] Close the bladder wall incision with a 4–0 synthetic absorbable suture.[70] Administer appropriate antibiotics 7 to 10 days postoperatively.[70]

Long-term cystotomy tube placement can lead to a urinary tract infection. The presence of infection may require tube removal. Antibiotics should always be chosen by culture and sensitivity of the urine to avoid bacterial resistance. Close monitoring of the patient is necessary to prevent self-removal of the tube as well. Most ferrets tolerate this procedure and the postoperative care without incident.[70]

Gastrotomy/Enterotomy

Indications

Young ferrets tend to ingest foreign objects, particularly rubber. Ferrets can also develop GI obstructions with trichobezoars (figure 18). Abdominal palpation and radiography may be inconclusive. For objects that result in obstruction, removal is necessary (see chapter 7). In the event that endoscopy is not available or appropriate, laparotomy is the treatment of choice.

Anatomy

Ferrets have a simple stomach with a well-developed pylorus. The small intestine is short with no distinguishing features between the jejunum and ileum. There is no cecum in the large intestine and no ileocecal valve between the small intestine and colon.[7]

Procedure

Place an IV or IO catheter and administer LRS at 25 ml/kg/hr. Administer preoperative analgesia (see chapter 5, Anesthesia). Aseptically prepare the ventral abdomen with the anesthetized patient in dorsal recumbency. Make a ventral midline incision from xiphoid to pubis. Examine the intestinal tract thoroughly. Foreign material can be found anywhere along the GI tract, from stomach to colon. Gently manipulate objects in the distal esophagus or proximal duodenum into the stomach for simple gastrotomy.[64] Gastrotomy, enterotomy, and intestinal resection are performed in the same way as in cats and dogs. If gastritis is suspected, take a full-thickness biopsy specimen before closing the gastrotomy site. Gastrotomy incisions are closed in a double layer, a simple continuous pattern with 4–0 absorbable synthetic monofilament, followed by an inverting layer.[42] Make enterotomy incisions longitudinally along the antimesenteric border of the intestine.[42] Close enterotomy incisions with 4–0 or 5–0 absorbable synthetic monofilament in a simple interrupted or simple continuous appositional pattern, with care to include all layers of the intestinal wall. Close linear incisions transversely to avoid strictures.[42] When all intestinal incisions are closed, cover the sites with omentum.[18] Change gloves and instruments and flush the abdomen with warm sterile saline before routine abdominal closure.

Postsurgical considerations

Withhold food and water 6 to 12 hours postoperatively. Treat with postoperative analgesics as needed. Continue IV or IO fluids until the ferret is eating. Liquid diets may be necessary for the first few meals (5 cc every 2 to 3 hours), although most ferrets recover uneventfully, eating on their own within 24 hours of surgery.[18] Introduce food as soon as possible to reduce ileus and adhesion formation. An increase in body temperature, vomiting, and abdominal tenderness indicate postoperative peritonitis. If a suppurative exudate develops, perform an intestinal resection and anastomosis or a serosal patching technique as necessary. Enterotomy sites may stricture after surgery, increasing the chance of future blockage.[64]

Insulinoma

Indications

This is one of the most common neoplasms in the ferret.[59] Surgical intervention consists of debulking the tumor, which is usually diffuse throughout the pancreas, with metastasis to the liver. Although it is not curative, it may lengthen the life span and improve the effectiveness of medical therapy. It is generally recommended for ferrets younger than 5 years of age and in otherwise good health. See chapter 7 for further information.

Anatomy

The pancreas is a V-shaped, elongated, and lobulated gland, with two arms connected by a body located close to the pylorus. The left lobe lies in the mesoduodenum dorsal to the visceral surface of the stomach. The longer right lobe follows the descending duodenum, then doubles back on itself, lying at the mesenteric root. The common pancreatic duct joins the bile duct, emptying into the duodenum at the major duodenal papilla 2.8 cm caudal to the cranial duodenal flexure.[7,42]

Procedure

Administer preanesthetic analgesics. Place an IV or IO catheter. In patients with severe clinical signs, begin fluid therapy with 2.5% dextrose in 0.45% saline 12 hours preoperatively. Support the ferret with 2.5% dextrose in 0.45% saline or 5% dextrose in water during surgery. Limit presurgical fasting to 3 to 4 hours. Aseptically prepare the ventral abdomen while the anesthetized patient is in dorsal recumbency. Make a ventral midline incision from xiphoid to pubis. Exteriorize the spleen, wrapping it in warm saline-moistened gauze. The pancreas will be visible in the greater omentum.[24] Gentle manipulation of the duodenum will reveal the ventral and dorsal aspects of the right lobe within the mesoduodenum.[42] Most commonly, multiple nodules will be present in the pancreas[54] (figure 19). Occasionally, only a single nodule will be seen.[64] Gently palpate the entire pancreas for the presence of nodules deep in the tissues. Distinct nodules can be removed via gentle blunt dissection.[64] Gelfoam (Upjohn, Kalamazoo, MI) or gentle pressure will provide hemostasis.[64] One study indicates that a combination of nodular excision with partial pancreatectomy increases the disease-free interval and survival time in the ferret.[71] Partial pancreatectomy is also an option in a patient with no visible or palpable nodules but clear clinical signs of disease. One limb of the pancreas is removed and submitted for histopathology to determine the presence of microscopic nodules.

Two techniques are available for partial pancreatectomy in the ferret. Take care to avoid compromising the vascular supply to the spleen (left lobe) or proximal duodenum (right lobe).[42] In the suture fracture technique, the lobes are gently dissected away from adjacent structures.[64] A single nonreactive absorbable suture is placed around that section of pancreas, crushing the tissue and ligating the ducts and vessels within.[64] Trim the section away from the suture for biopsy.[64] Close the defect in the omentum or mesentery to prevent visceral entrapment.[42] In the dissection and ligation techniques, the vessels and ductules are ligated with hemostatic clips or fine absorbable monofilament suture as they are exposed during the dissection.[42] Transection distal to the sutures allows removal of the tissue.[42]

Metastasis to the liver, spleen, mesenteric lymph nodes, and other abdominal structures can occur. If this is noted, resect and biopsy the affected tissues. Flush the surgical site with warmed sterile saline to remove pancreatic enzymes and surgical debris before routine closure of the abdomen.

Postsurgical considerations

Administer postoperative analgesics as needed. Monitor blood and urine glucose levels immediately after surgery and every 6 to 12 hours for the next 48 hours. When the blood glucose level is normal and the ferret is eating, discontinue fluid therapy. Begin adjunct medical therapy for patients that do not become normoglycemic within 1 to 2 days postoperatively (see chapter 7). Offer a bland, high-protein, low-carbohydrate diet in small frequent amounts within 12 hours of recovery. Pancreatitis is rare in ferrets, even after pancreatic surgery. Transient diabetes has been seen postoperatively but usually resolves without treatment. (For more information see chapter 7, Pancreas.) Monitor blood glucose 10 to 14 days postoperatively and every 1 to 3 months thereafter.[42,64]

Orchiectomy

Indications

The majority of male ferrets in the United States are castrated before sale to the public. Intact male ferrets tend to be more aggressive, less social, and have a distinctly strong and musky body odor, especially when sexually active. Neutering removes most of this odor and decreases aggressive tendencies. Castration also prevents testicular neoplasia, which has been reported in the ferret.[72] Surgery should be performed between 6 and 12 months of age. Cryptorchidism can occur unilaterally or bilaterally. The retained testes can be located within the inguinal canal or the abdomen, requiring a laparotomy for removal.

Anatomy

The ferret testes are located caudoventrally in the scrotal sac. They show a significant enlargement in size during the reproductive season.[5,7]

Procedure

Orchiectomy in ferrets can be performed as in dogs or cats, as either an open or closed procedure. Two procedures will be described. Preoperative butorphanol for analgesia aids recovery. For the first procedure, place the anesthetized ferret in dorsal recumbency and septically prepare the prescrotal area as in the dog. Make a single prescrotal incision. Exteriorize each testicle, double ligating the spermatic cord and testicular vessels in an open or closed fashion, as the surgeon prefers. Allow the stumps to retract into the incision. Perform routine subcuticular closure with 4–0 or 5–0 absorbable suture. Skin sutures are unnecessary.

The second procedure is similar to that performed in the cat. With the anesthetized ferret in dorsal recumbency, shave or pluck the scrotal sack. After aseptic preparation, make two longitudinal scrotal incisions, removing the testicles for double ligation of the vessel and cord, either open or closed, with 4–0 absorbable suture. The scrotal incisions are left open to heal, as in the cat.

Postsurgical considerations

There are few postsurgical problems with ferret castration. Recovery is usually uneventful, and the patient is released the same day. Rarely, postoperative hemorrhage due to slipped ligatures or hemorrhaging gubernacular attachments is seen. Exploration of the scrotum reveals the problem, which is resolved with appropriate hemostasis.

Orthopedics

Indications

As with any companion animal, fractures and dislocations caused by accidental injury can occur. The same orthopedic principles for correction used in other small animals apply to ferrets.

Procedure

In all cases of trauma, shock should be treated first. When the animal's condition is stabilized and all bleeding controlled, perform a thorough orthopedic and neurologic examination. Open fractures should be covered and supported. It is important to keep the patient quiet and administer analgesics until anesthetic risk is at a minimum. At that time, appropriate fracture or dislocation repair can be performed.

It is important for the surgeon to remember the size of the patient and choose a method of repair accordingly. Splints, pins, plates, and external fixators all have their place, depending on the type of injury.[73] In the event of unrepairable trauma, amputation is well tolerated. The procedure is the same as that in a cat.

Postsurgical considerations

As in any fracture repair, the possibilities of delayed union, nonunion, and malunion are always present.[73] These are caused by infection, lack of blood supply, poor immobilization, and unequal stresses on the bone.[73] Correction of the cause may lead to proper bone healing. Treat osteomyelitis with appropriate antibiotics after culture and sensitivity testing of the fracture site. If proper alignment does not occur, cage rest may lead to functional but misaligned healing of the bones. These pets tolerate such limitations very well and adapt to their environment quickly. Amputation is also an option.

Ovariohysterectomy

Indications

The majority of female ferrets in the United States are spayed before sale to the public. If they are not to be used for breeding, they should be spayed by 4 to 6 months of age or within 2 weeks of their first estrus. Because they are induced ovulators, estrus continues until breeding occurs. If the estrous cycle is not interrupted, the level of estrogens can cause suppression of the bone marrow to the point of fatal aplastic anemia in 50% of jills.[29] Other indications for ovariohysterectomy (OVH) include pyometra and reproductive tract neoplasia. Abdominal exploratory examination for ovarian remnant removal is indicated in ferrets younger than 2 years with signs of estrus, regardless of OVH history.

Anatomy

The ferret has a bicornate uterus, with a short body fused just cranial to the cervix.[7]

Procedure

Regardless of the duration of signs of estrus, obtain a CBC and platelet count prior to surgery to detect anemia. Transfusion is indicated when the packed cell volume (PCV) is less than 20%.[18] Administer IV or IO fluid therapy and transfusion preoperatively to stabilize the patient.

The OVH procedure in ferrets is similar to that in cats. Aseptically prepare the ventral abdomen of the dorsally recumbent, anesthetized patient. A 2- to 3-cm ventral midline incision extending caudally from the umbilicus gives access to the ovaries and uterus. Abdominal fat deposits can make identification of the ovaries and vasculature difficult.[64] Be cautious of the ureters during ligation, because they lie near the ovaries.[64] Exteriorize the uterus and ovaries with a spay hook or careful digital manipulation.[54] Double ligate the ovarian vessels with 4–0 absorbable synthetic suture.[64] The suspensory ligament is easily torn to allow double ligation of the uterine body just cranial to the cervix.[54] Remove the uterus and ovaries via transection, and close the abdomen routinely. If skin sutures are used, remove in 7 to 10 days.

If ovarian remnants are suspected, make a ventral midline incision from xiphoid to pubis to explore the abdomen. Ovarian remnants are usually found caudolateral to the caudal pole of the kidney but may be anywhere in the abdomen, especially in the mesenteric fat.[64] Ligate any vessels attached to the remnant. Bluntly dissect the remnants, followed by Gelfoam (Upjohn, Kalamazoo, MI) or digital pressure for hemostasis. Thorough examination of the adrenal glands is indicated in any spayed ferret with an enlarged vulva, regardless of age. Close the abdomen routinely. Remove skin sutures in 7 to 10 days. Perform histopathology on remnants, as in some cases they can be neoplastic.[44]

Postsurgical considerations

Recovery from this surgery is usually uneventful. If the patient was showing signs of anemia before surgery, monitor the red blood cell (RBC) count, PCV, and platelet count frequently until all values return to normal. In ovarian remnant removal, the vulva should return to normal in 1 to 5 days.[64]

Splenectomy

Indications

Splenectomy is recommended for patients with severe splenomegaly, splenic interference with normal abdominal function, splenic neoplasia, or an irregular or lumpy spleen.[24,42] Splenic biopsy is recommended preoperatively, as partial splenectomy is preferable to complete removal of the organ.[42]

Anatomy

The spleen is a crescent-shaped, gray-brown organ firmly attached to the stomach and liver by the gastrosplenic ligament, part of the greater omentum.[7]

Procedure

Place an IV or IO catheter and administer LRS or saline at 25 ml/kg/hr. Administer preoperative analgesics. Place the anesthetized ferret in dorsal recumbency and aseptically prepare the ventral abdomen. Make a ventral midline incision from xiphoid to pubis. Exteriorize the spleen.

For a partial splenectomy in nonneoplastic conditions, removal of the caudal portion is least likely to cause vascular compromise to the stomach.[42] Double ligate or hemoclip the vessels supplying the chosen portion of the spleen and transect at the hilus.[42] After several minutes, a line of demarcation will be seen between the viable portion of the spleen and the section deprived of blood.[42] Pinch the spleen at this demarcation between thumb and forefinger, milking the parenchyma

oward the ischemic portion.[42] Clamp the flattened portion with a for-
eps or 23-cm Kocher intestinal forceps.[24] Transect the spleen distal to
he clamp. Suture the cut surface with 4–0 absorbable synthetic in a
ontinuous pattern or place surgical staples.[42] Alternatively, place mat-
ress sutures through the parietal and visceral surfaces of the spleen
long the line of demarcation.[42] Use digital pressure, Gelfoam
Upjohn, Kalamazoo, MI), or Surgicel (Johnson & Johnson Healthcare
ystems, Piscataway, NJ) for hemostasis after clamp removal.[42]

Perform a total splenectomy by double ligating or using surgical clips
n the vessels at the hilus, beginning at the caudal end.[42] Transect the
essels between ligatures.[42]

Postoperative considerations

Administer postoperative analgesics as needed. The spleen in an
soflurane-anesthetized ferret sequesters a significant amount of red
lood cells.[24] Monitor PCV postoperatively until the values return to
ormal, administering blood transfusions as needed.[24] Ischemic pan-
reatitis can result from inappropriate ligation of the vessels during
plenectomy.[42]

Vasectomy

Indications

Vasectomized males are used by ferret breeders to bring intact females
out of season.

Anatomy

The ferret testes are located caudoventrally in the scrotal sac. The def-
erent duct is carried within the spermatic cord on the ventral surface of
he testis.[7]

Procedure

Administer preoperative analgesia. Place the anesthetized patient in dorsal recumbency. Aseptically prepare the skin cranially and laterally to and including the scrotum. Gently retract the scrotum. Make a 1- to 1.5-cm incision craniolaterally to the scrotal sac.[74] Bluntly dissect the underlying tissues to reveal the spermatic cord. Enter the vaginal tunic and isolate the vas deferens, a thin opaque ribbon of tissue.[74] Clamp and ligate the vas deferens in two places, 3 to 4 mm apart.[74] Excise the section of the duct and remove the clamps.[74] Skin closure is at the surgeon's discretion; internal or external sutures and cyanoacrylate are all viable choices. Repeat sequence on the second testicle. Remove sutures in 7 to 10 days.

Postsurgical considerations

Surgical recovery is usually uneventful. Administer postoperative analgesia as needed. Whereas intact male ferrets normally have distinct seasons of sexual activity, in the author's experience (Purcell) vasectomized males may become sexually active year-round.

Diagnosis and
Disease

Introduction

The ferret suffers from a wide variety of disorders. As these animals have increased in popularity as pets, more interest has been taken in studying these disease problems, and new information is coming out almost daily. A network of practitioners knowledgeable in ferret medicine and available as advisors and sounding boards is invaluable. It is equally important to keep up with current treatments and techniques via conferences, wet laboratories, textbooks, periodicals, and the Internet. Some of the information contained in this book may change in a short period of time; therefore, this discussion is aimed at giving the practitioner a start and a direction to the diagnostic thought process, but it is not meant to be the definitive answer in all cases. Good critical thinking skills and adherence to sound medical practice are helpful in handling ferrets and modifying existing diagnostic skills and techniques.

Cardiovascular System

Introduction

The ferret heart is found between the sixth and eighth ribs, more caudal than that of cats and dogs.[7] There is a normal pronounced sinus arrhythmia on auscultation, and a transient bradycardia may be noted.[31]

Heart disease is common in ferrets older than 3 years. It is important to screen for abnormalities early, to determine the normal parameters for each ferret as it ages (figure 20). Radiography shows heart enlargement in many ferrets, but there is no evidence of clinical disease when evaluated by ultrasonography and electrocardiography. Yearly thoracic radiographs of ferrets older than 3 years help screen for potential problems.

Clinical signs of cardiac disease can include hind limb weakness, anorexia, weight loss, elevated respiratory rate or dyspnea, lethargy, vomiting, ascites, and, rarely, coughing.[31,44,75] A physical examination can reveal hypothermia, cyanosis, prolonged capillary refill time, weak or irregular pulses, tachypnea with or without open-mouth breathing, jugular pulses, a murmur or arrhythmia on auscultation, and muffled heart or lung sounds.[31,44,75] Lung sounds may include crackles and/or wheezes. Hepatomegaly is secondary to circulatory disturbances. Concurrent disease is common, so all physical abnormalities should be noted carefully.[31,75]

The differential diagnosis for a patient with suspected cardiac disease includes cardiomyopathy, valve disorders, and heartworm as well as noncardiac disease such as lymphoma, insulinoma, and gastrointestinal foreign body. Thoracic radiographs and echocardiography aid in distinguishing cardiac abnormalities. An electrocardiogram (ECG) is valuable in detecting arrhythmias and conduction disorders.[47] A complete blood cell (CBC) count, serum biochemistry screen, and abdominal radiographs are recommended for detection of underlying disease. If thoracic fluid is present, thoracocentesis with cytology is indicated.

Cardiomyopathy

The most common cardiac disease of the ferret is cardiomyopathy.[44] Although both dilative and hypertrophic forms are seen, the majority of references cite the dilative form as the more common.[31,44,75] The etiology of cardiomyopathy in the ferret is unknown. There may be a connection between dietary deficiency of taurine and the dilative form of cardiomyopathy as seen in the cat, but this relationship has not been proven.[47,76]

The clinical presentation of a ferret with dilative cardiomyopathy is that of a lethargic animal 3 years of age or older with a history of weight loss, anorexia, and respiratory distress.[31] Auscultation can reveal tachycardia, a systolic murmur, moist rales, and muffled heart and lung sounds.[31] Hypothermia, ascites, and hind limb weakness are noted on physical examination.[31] Cardiomyopathy is diagnosed on the basis of radiographic and ultrasonographic findings (figure 21). On the plain radiograph, the first sign of cardiomegaly is loss of the radiolucent area between the heart and sternum, so that the heart appears to be resting directly on the sternum. Pulmonary edema or pleural effusion may be present.[31] Abdominal radiographs may indicate hepatomegaly, splenomegaly, and/or ascites.[31] Electrocardiographic results are variable.[31] Ultrasound examination is the most accurate way to differentiate between the forms of cardiomyopathy.[76] Dilative cardiomyopathy presents as left atrial enlargement and right ventricular dilation on ultrasonic examination.[31,76] Doppler echocardiography usually shows mitral valve regurgitation and occasionally tricuspid valve regurgitation.[31,76] Decreased aortic flow may also be noted.[31]

Early cases of dilated cardiomyopathy may be controlled with the use of diuretics such as furosemide. Digoxin improves cardiac contractility but has known toxic effects in mammals.[47,76] Ferrets are sensitive to the balanced vasodilators, such as enalapril (Enacard, Merck & Co., Whitehouse Station, NJ) or 2% nitroglycerin cream, which can cause lethargy. Patients need to be monitored carefully and dosages adjusted as needed.[31] In ferrets with clinical signs despite the use of diuretics, and with owners who decline further diagnostics to differentiate dilative and hypertrophic disease, enalapril is the drug of choice.[18] A low-salt diet and decreased exercise are also recommended but may be difficult to implement.[31] Therapy should be monitored with regular chemistry panels, blood digoxin levels, and ultrasonography.[75] The long-term prognosis for patients with dilated cardiomyopathy is guarded to fair.[31,44] If diagnosed early and given the proper therapy, many of these ferrets can have a good quality of life for many months.[44]

Hypertrophic cardiomyopathy has been reported in ferrets, but a complete clinical picture has not yet been presented.[75] The clinical presentation can be normal, include vague complaints of lethargy, or present as a sudden death.[31,44] Physical examination may detect a systolic murmur or arrythmia (often tachycardia), but some patients are asymptomatic.[31,44] Subclinical disease is often discovered 24 hours postoperatively, with a sudden decompensation.[44] Cardiomegaly is not a consistent finding on thoracic radiographs.[44] Ultrasonic examination reveals thickened left ventricular walls and interventricular septum.[31] Heart function may be normal or hyperdynamic.[31] Doppler echocardiography usually shows mitral regurgitation.[31] Treatment focuses on improving heart function while decreasing congestion. Beta-blockers such as propranolol or atenolol and calcium channel antagonists such as diltiazem reduce the heart rate, improve filling time, and cause myocardial relaxation. When these are combined with diuretics as described earlier, the disease can be controlled, but the prognosis is guarded, depending on the individual response to treatment.[44,75,77]

Valvular disease

Valvular disease usually occurs in ferrets 3 years of age and older. Clinical signs of this disease are variable. The first indication is usually a holosystolic murmur on the left.[31] Moist rales may be auscultated as well.[31] Radiographic and ECG evidence is also variable.[31] Echocardiography gives a definitive diagnosis, revealing left or right atrial enlargement, corresponding mild ventricular dilation, and valvular regurgitation.[31] Heart function is normal or increased.[31] Initial treatment with furosemide and enalapril reduces the heart load and congestion.[31] As the disease progresses, especially if supraventricular arrhythmias develop, add digoxin to increase cardiac contractility.[31,75] The prognosis is guarded.

Heartworm disease

Ferrets are susceptible to heartworm disease in endemic areas of the country. The ferret is naturally infected with *Dirofilaria immitis*, and because of the small size of the heart even the presence of one adult worm can cause serious cardiac obstructive disease.[31] Clinical signs can be vague and include dyspnea, anorexia, melena, lethargy, occasional coughing, and sudden death.[76,78] On physical examination, pulmonary congestion, ascites, and a grade II to III heart murmur may be noted.[76,78] A peripheral eosinophilia may be present. Pulmonary congestion and/or pleural effusion with right-sided heart enlargement can be seen on thoracic radiography and must be differentiated from other cardiac disease.[31,79] Pruning of vessels and right ventricular enlargement may also be present radiographically.[76] Dr. Deborah Kemmerer reported accurate results using the CITE Snap heartworm test (IDEXX Laboratories, Inc., Westbrook, ME) to diagnose this disease.[30] Ultrasonography can also be used for diagnosis, showing the presence of adult worms in the right ventricle or vena cava, but results have not been consistent.[44] Other direct or occult heartworm tests have proved unreliable in the ferret. Ferrets usually do not produce circulating microfilaria when infected naturally.

Dr. Kemmerer has treated heartworm-infected ferrets with an approximately 70% success rate.[30] Thromboembolisms may occur up to 8 months after treatment, so concurrent treatment with corticosteroids is recommended. Give caparsolate (2.2 mg/kg IV) in four injections at 12-hour intervals via cephalic IV catheter. On the first day of caparsolate treatment, start prednisone (0.5–1.0 mg per ferret per day). Continue prednisone therapy until a CITE test is negative, then taper the dose until it is discontinued.[30] During and after the treatment regimen, the ferret should be confined in a cage without exercise or play.[77] A follow-up CITE heartworm test is done at 3 months and repeated monthly until negative. Heartworm prevention should be started 1 month after the negative test results.

Melarsamine hydrochloride (Immiticide, Rhone-Merieux, Athens, GA) should not be used as a possible treatment. This medication kills the worms too quickly, leading to fatal emboli.[80]

Prevention is the best way to avoid this disease in the ferret. Give ivermectin orally on a monthly basis during the heartworm season. The ivermectin dosage recommended by the American Heartworm Society for ferrets is 0.006 mg/kg monthly.[77] Use the injectable form orally (Ivomec, Merck, Whitehouse Station, NJ) or the tablet form designed for the feline patient (Heartgard, Merck). Ferrets should not be housed outdoors in endemic areas unless receiving preventive therapy.

Endocrine System

Adrenal glands

The majority of the generalized alopecias seen in neutered ferrets 2 years of age and older are caused by adrenal-associated endocrinopathy.[59] In the American ferret this appears to be a primary adrenal disease, with no evidence to date of pituitary involvement. This disease can be caused by adrenocortical hyperplasia or neoplasms, most commonly cortical adenoma or cortical adenocarcinoma.[29,69,72] Metastasis can occur.[49,69] Pheochromocytoma has been reported to affect the area cranial to the right kidney and involve the vena cava but does not lead to adrenal-associated endocrinopathy.[60]

The etiology is unknown, but factors such as early neutering of ferrets (before 6 weeks of age), genetic predisposition, and exposure to unnatural photoperiods (i.e., not being kept in natural lighting conditions) have been implicated by various authorities.[60] The authors have noted through communications with practitioners in Europe, Australia, and New Zealand, where adrenal-associated endocrinopathy is rare, that there are significant differences in husbandry. In non-U.S. countries, ferrets are usually neutered after sexual maturity, housed outdoors under natural lighting conditions, not inbred to acquire fancy colors, and fed a natural or nonprocessed diet.

Adrenal-associated endocrinopathy in ferrets is entirely different from the corresponding disease syndrome in the dog (Cushing's disease). In ferrets, estrogen precursors such as androstenedione, 17-hydroxypro-gesterone, estradiol, and dehydroepiandrosterone sulfate (DHEAS) are often elevated.[46] Cortisol levels are not affected by this disease. Signs of adrenal neoplasia are usually seen in ferrets 2 years of age or older and of either sex. The most common presenting clinical sign is bilater-ally symmetrical alopecia, usually starting at the hind end and progressing forward on the body[49] (figure 22). The history may reveal that the ferret had a previous episode of hair loss and then regrew the hair spontaneously.[46] There is commonly mild to severe pruritus with or without small scabs and excoriations.[81] Intense pruritus without alopecia is a rarer variation.[81] Atrophy of abdominal and hind limb musculature can occur, leading to hind limb weakness and a potbellied appearance.[49] Lethargy may be noted, most often described by clients as increased sleeping habits.[49] Both males and females may have an increase in sebaceous secretions and body odor as if they were still reproductively intact. Approximately 50% of spayed females present with vulvar enlargement with or without a mucoid discharge[29,46,49] (figure 23). Males may become aggressive and display mounting behavior.[46,49] In addition, males can present with signs of dysuria or acute urinary obstruction due to prostatic enlargement or paraurethral cysts.[46,81] Normal ferret adrenal glands are not easily palpated. On physical examination of a ferret with adrenal disease, one or both of the adrenals may be palpably enlarged.[81] Splenomegaly and enlarged mesenteric lymph nodes are a common incidental finding on palpa-tion.[81]

The diagnosis of adrenal-associated endocrinopathy is based on his-tory, clinical signs, and physical examination findings. Usually, surgical exploration confirms the diagnosis. CBC count results are generally unremarkable, although rarely mild anemia and thrombocy-topenia are found.[49,63] The biochemistry panel is also within normal limits, although occasionally serum glutamic-pyruvic transaminase

(SGPT) is elevated.[63,82] A urinalysis may indicate cystitis or prostatic abnormalities by the presence of pyuria with squamous epithelial cells.[29] If clinical signs are vague, an androgen panel can be obtained to detect elevated androgen and estrogen levels.[83,84] (See Resources, Medical Information, at the back of the book.) In ferrets with adrenal-associated endocrinopathy, DHEAS, 17-hydroxyprogesterone, androgesterone, testosterone, and/or estradiol is usually elevated.[46] As cortisol is not affected in this disorder, dexamethasone suppression tests and adrenocorticotropic hormone (ACTH) stimulation are nondiagnostic.[82] Radiographs seldom detect these tumors because of the small size and lack of mineralization of the adrenal glands but are recommended to screen for cardiac disease and other abnormalities.[82] Ultrasonography can detect larger tumors and is particularly useful in the diagnosis of concurrent disease, such as paraurethral cysts, renal or liver disease, cardiac abnormalities, and other neoplasms present in the abdomen.[82] A computed tomographic scan also reveals adrenal gland abnormalities.

Adrenal-associated endocrinopathy can be treated by surgical removal of the gland(s) and/or medical management. In addition, the abdominal exploratory examination is a valuable diagnostic tool in the ferret because of the high incidence of concurrent neoplasia (e.g., insulinoma or lymphoma). (See chapter 6, Adrenalectomy.)

Postoperative histological examination of adrenal glands from clinically ill patients has found normal tissue, nodular hyperplasia, adrenocortical carcinoma, adrenocortical adenoma, pheochromocytoma, and myelolipoma.[59] Cysts have been seen in association with right adrenal tumors.[49] In one study, 100% of the neutered males exhibiting sexual behavior were diagnosed with carcinoma at biopsy.[49]

In cases in which surgery is not an option because of the advanced age of the patient, concurrent disease, or lack of funds, medical management can be considered. The most commonly used treatment is *o*, *p*-DDD or mitotane (Lysodren, Bristol-Myers Squibb Oncology,

Princeton, NJ). Mitotane selectively destroys the zona fasciculata and zona reticularis of the adrenal cortex.[85] Unfortunately, it is frequently unsuccessful in reducing clinical signs in ferrets.[82] Cases of adrenal cortical adenocarcinoma are generally unresponsive.[82] Adrenal hyperplasia and cortical adenomas have more promise for treatment, and in some cases o, p-DDD has been completely palliative for 1 year or longer. However, it is difficult to assess the true efficacy of mitotane in these cases, as adrenal disease can regress spontaneously without treatment. It has been shown that o, p-DDD effectively reduces blood cortisol levels in ferrets; if the ferret has concurrent insulinoma, treatment with o, p-DDD can aggravate this condition.

The treatment protocol varies according to the patient. Mitotane has very low toxicity in the ferret. It does not affect bone marrow, so serial CBC counts are not necessary. Its primary side effects are gastrointestinal (e.g., nausea, vomiting). Treatment should be postponed for 4 weeks in the event of severe vomiting and restarted at half-dose.[58] Divide the mitotane tablets into 50-mg portions, mix with cornstarch as a filler, and place in small gelatin capsules. The patient is dosed at 50 mg per ferret once daily for 7 days, then every third day for 8 to 12 weeks. (The more exact dose is 50 mg/kg body weight, but it is difficult to divide the powdered tablet accurately.) The capsule must be given whole and cannot be mixed with other substances because this may reduce its efficacy. Give prednisone (0.5–1.0 mg/kg every 12 hours) concurrently.[69] Therapy results can be monitored with the ACTH stimulation test after the first week of treatment (loading dose). Administer ACTH (1 U/kg IM) and measure serum cortisol at 0 and 60 minutes.[86] If there is no decrease in cortisol or response to therapy at the end of 12 weeks, treatment is discontinued. The author (Brown) has tried the therapy every other day for several weeks with no ill effect, and therapy should be altered as needed. If there is a response of hair regrowth or reduction of vulvar swelling, then the dosage is reduced when the patient appears normal for at least 2 weeks. The patient should be weaned from medication gradually. If signs recur, the protocol is started again but continued for life, giving mitotane at least once a week. Vulvar swelling and hair regrowth can occur spontaneously in this disease, regardless of treatment, increasing the difficulty of evaluating the success of treatment. Attempts to use ketoconazole to treat this disease have been unsuccessful.[82]

In males with urinary obstruction caused by paraurethral cysts, where surgery is unavailable, medical treatment with flutamide has been successful in some cases. Dr. Karen Rosenthal has performed trials on ferrets with flutamide, a pure androgen blocker used in human males with benign prostatic hyperplasia.[63] Flutamide (10 mg/kg every 12 to 24 hours PO) is administered to decrease prostatic tissue enlargement and paraurethral cysts.[18,63] Urinary obstruction must be alleviated before therapy (see chapter 6, Surgery), and treatment with flutamide is lifelong.

In pets that exhibit concurrent adrenal disease and insulinoma, where quality of life is the only consideration, some practitioners are using megestrol acetate to resolve clinical signs.[87] Results are mixed, and this protocol deserves further study. Megestrol acetate is a synthetic progestin with significant antiestrogen and glucocorticoid activity, which suppresses adrenal function.[88] It also interferes with the conversion of testosterone to dihydrotestosterone, a hormone that promotes prostatic hyperplasia.[89] The glucocorticoid effects of this medication increase blood glucose, decreasing the need for separate medication to treat concurrent insulinoma. Use this drug with care, as it can precipitate pyometra in intact females and has led to diabetes mellitus and adrenal atrophy in cats.[88] The current recommended dose is 1 mg every 24 hours PO for 3 days, then 1 mg every 3 to 4 days, gradually tapering the dose to the minimum clinically effective.[87] Clinical response includes partial or complete hair regrowth and weight gain.[87]

Adrenal-associated endocrinopathy tends to be a very slowly progressive disease, and ferrets may have a good quality of life for 2 to years after diagnosis without treatment. Alopecia may be intermittent. Use emollient skin oil sprays to treat dry or pruritic skin and use soft bedding. Aplastic anemia is rarely a problem but can occur in either sex. These animals may benefit from anabolic steroids and vitamin supplementation, although steroids are contraindicated in the presence of aplastic anemia. Even untreated, ferrets with adrenal tumors can have a good quality of life for several years.

Pancreas—diabetes mellitus

Diabetes is rare in the ferret, usually seen as a transient condition after surgical removal of insulinomas.[82] (See chapter 6, Insulinoma.) One suggested etiology is a diet heavy in carbohydrates, particularly sugar-coated foods.[18] Clinical signs include severe lethargy, weakness, polyuria, polydipsia, and weight loss.[82,90] A CBC count is usually unremarkable. Dehydration and ketosis may be seen with chronic or severe disease. Urinalysis can also reveal an active sediment related to a secondary cystitis. Diagnosis is based on persistent hyperglycemia (glucose > 300 mg/dl) with glucosuria.[82] Use insulin levels to differentiate diabetes mellitus from a glucagonoma. Insulin levels need to be determined at a laboratory that has calibration for ferret blood insulin levels. Low insulin levels are indicative of diabetes mellitus.[82] Normal or high insulin concentrations can indicate an insulin-resistant state or glucagonoma.[82] Radiography and ultrasonography are nondiagnostic for diabetes.

Treatment follows the basic feline protocols. Like cats, ferrets can be difficult to regulate.[18,82] One recommended protocol begins with NPH (neutral protamine Hagadorn) at 0.1 U per ferret every 12 hours as a starting dose, increasing until an effective dose is reached.[82] Serial blood glucose tests and urine monitoring for ketonuria and glucosuria are performed in the hospital. When the blood levels are consistently below 200 mg/dl, the ferret can be discharged to the owners with instructions to continue twice daily dosing at the current in-hospital rate, with at-home monitoring of the urine for glucose to titrate the optimal dose per day. Ultralente insulin can be used to attempt once-daily dosing at home. Instructions for at-home monitoring are as follows: if no glucose is present in the urine, no insulin is given; if trace glucose is found, the dose does not change; if a large amount of glucose is found in the urine, the dose is increased slightly.[82] Oral forms of insulin are not useful in the ferret.[18]

The prognosis for ferrets with transient diabetes related to surgery is good, as the hyperglycemia usually resolves without treatment in 1 to 2 weeks.[82] In ferrets with non–surgery-related diabetes or nonresolving hyperglycemia, the prognosis is variable, pending the ability to regulate the blood glucose levels.[82] In ferrets presenting with an initial blood glucose greater than 500 mg/dl, the prognosis for response to treatment is poor.[29]

Pancreas—insulinoma

Insulinoma, or pancreatic beta cell tumor, occurs with about the same frequency as adrenal neoplasia, and the conditions are often concurrent.[59] Hypoglycemia is the primary problem in insulinoma.[8,82] Insulinoma can affect both male and female ferrets 2 years of age or older. The etiology of the disease is unknown, but factors such as genetic predisposition and a diet too high in carbohydrates have been considered. As in the case of adrenal neoplasia, veterinarians in Europe, New Zealand, and Australia do not report insulinoma to be a major problem in their ferret patients. In these countries, raw whole prey items are the predominant diet, rather than processed foods. In England, where processed food use is increasing among ferret owners, several practitioners have reported a rise in insulinoma cases.[18]

These tumors produce high levels of insulin, driving glucose out of the bloodstream and into the cells at a rapid rate.[91] As the blood glucose level drops, the brain becomes deprived of energy, which impairs normal function.[91] The muscles also become weak.[91] Early in the disease, weight loss may be the only abnormality.[82,92] The body responds with several counterregulatory mechanisms to bring the blood glucose level back to normal. Therefore, the signs of insulinoma are intermittent, may be subtle and short-lived, and resolve without treatment early in the disease.[91] A ferret experiencing a hypoglycemic attack may be observed to stare blankly into space for a few seconds to minutes, unaware of its surroundings, or exhibit hind limb weakness or lethargy. The pet may salivate and paw at the mouth, probably an indication of nausea. Clients often present these ferrets as an emergency, suspecting a foreign body in the mouth. Vomiting and sudden collapse are often noted. As the disease progresses, the periods of weakness and lethargy become more pronounced in intensity, duration, and frequency. Eventually the signs progress to seizures, coma, and death.

The diagnosis is based on clinical signs and the demonstration of a low fasting blood glucose level.[91] The pet should be fasted for 4 to 6 hours; a longer fast could result in a serious hypoglycemic attack. Insulinoma is such a common problem in ferrets that a fasting blood glucose level is recommended at least annually for all ferrets 3 years of age or older. The normal fasting glucose level for a ferret is approximately 90 to 125 mg/dl.[82] A fasting glucose level of 70 mg/dl or lower should raise suspicion of insulinoma.[82] Ferrets with glucose levels between 70 and 85 mg/dl should have the fasting glucose retested as well as an insulin level tested. Each laboratory should determine a baseline normal range for ferret insulin levels. Ferrets with blood glucose levels of 65 mg/dl or lower may show normal blood insulin levels, as seen in the dog, so insulin levels should not be used as a diagnostic tool in these cases.[91] If a ferret is showing signs of insulinoma but the blood glucose level remains high, it may be necessary to test the animal on more than one occasion and at different times of the day to detect a low blood glucose. CBC counts are usually unremarkable, but may reveal leukocytosis, neutrophilia, and monocytosis.[82] Blood chemistry panels may indicate increases in alanine aminotransferase (ALT) and aspartate aminotransferase (AST) levels, along with hypoglycemia.[82] Radiography is nondiagnostic for insulinoma. Ultrasonography is not diagnostic for insulinoma but may reveal metastatic lesions in the liver or spleen.

In the event of uncontrollable hypoglycemic episodes, continuous seizures, or collapse, admit the ferret for hospital treatment. Administer 50% dextrose as a slow IV bolus until the patient responds. If there is no response, treat for shock with IV fluids and corticosteroids and maintain a continuous infusion of 5% dextrose.[82] A rapid increase in blood glucose concentration can have a stimulating effect on the insulinoma, causing a rebound release of insulin and severe hypoglycemia.[82] When the patient is conscious, start feeding a high-protein, high-fat diet and begin prednisone therapy as needed. Monitor these patients carefully for 1 to 2 days. If necessary, anticonvulsant therapy with diazepam, titrated to effect, can be initiated until blood glucose levels are corrected.[82]

Management of insulinoma in the ferret can be surgical, medical, or a combination of both. The treatment regimen is unique for each ferret, depending on age, concurrent disease, severity of clinical signs, and owner preference. Because of the diffuse nature of this disease, no treatment is curative.

Surgery is not curative but rather is a debulking procedure, as insulinoma is usually found throughout the pancreas, has a high rate of recurrence, and can metastasize to other tissues (most notably the liver and spleen). However, surgical debulking can confirm the diagnosis, identify concurrent disease, prolong the patient's life, and decrease the need for postoperative medication.[82] Surgery can be performed repeatedly, but most clients prefer to control the disease with diet and medication after the first exploratory operation. See chapter 6, Insulinoma, for surgical procedures and postoperative care.

Medical management of insulinoma includes dietary control and medication. Attempt dietary control before medical therapy unless the patient is already exhibiting moderate to severe clinical signs. Give the ferret frequent meals with a high-quality animal protein and high fat content. High-quality cat foods, ferret foods, raw or cooked meat, cooked egg, and fermented dairy products such as cottage cheese and plain yogurt are suitable. Strained-meat baby foods, a/d (Hill's Pet Products, Topeka, KS), or a liquid high-protein diet can be used for treats or during periods when the pet is anorectic but should not make up the entire diet. Avoid the use of foods or treats high in sugar or carbohydrates, such as canine or feline semimoist diets, cookies, cakes, cereals, or dried fruit, which stimulate the release of insulin and aggravation of clinical signs. Brewer's yeast is a rich source of chromium, which is known as the glucose tolerance factor (GTF). Chromium is involved in the metabolism of glucose, and it helps to stabilize blood sugar and insulin levels in humans. Dr. Brown has noted that clients report an improvement in their pet's overall energy level when brewer's yeast is added to the diet. Use ¼ teaspoon of brewer's yeast powder sprinkled over the food or mixed with a protein snack twice daily.[18] Advise owners to keep honey or corn syrup on hand to administer in case of a severe hypoglycemic crisis. If the pet is unable to swallow, a mixture of warm water and honey can be rubbed on the gums and will revive the animal in 10 to 30 minutes. More of the mixture can be dripped into the mouth when the pet is conscious. As soon as the pet is completely alert, it is important to give a protein or high-fat meal or snack to prevent another hypoglycemic attack.

When diet no longer controls the signs (usually when the fasting glucose level is 50 mg/dl or below), medical therapy is instituted and continued for life. Corticosteroids are used to promote hepatic gluconeogenesis and inhibit cellular affinity for insulin.[91] Use prednisone (0.10 mg/kg PO every 12–24 hours initially) and increase the dosage gradually to control clinical signs. Doses up to 2 mg/kg PO every 12 hours have been reported.[82] Avoid using unnecessarily high doses of corticosteroids to prevent iatrogenic Cushing's disease. Avoid liquid medications compounded with alcohol to avoid unwanted side effects.[82] Diazoxide, a benzothiadiazide diuretic, is a useful adjunctive therapy to corticosteroids. Diazoxide primarily inhibits insulin secretion but also stimulates hepatic gluconeogenesis.[91] Diazoxide alone rarely controls clinical signs, but it is useful for reducing the amount of glucocorticoids needed and thus reducing the potential corticosteroid side effects. Give diazoxide (5–10 mg/kg PO every 12 hours) and reduce the prednisone dose if possible.[82] Diazoxide can be increased (up to 60 mg/kg divided every 8–12 hours) if necessary to control clinical signs.[82] The main drawback of the use of diazoxide is the expense. Ferrets can live for 1 to 3 years after diagnosis of insulinoma with a combination of surgery, dietary management, and medication.

Thyroid

Thyroid disorders are uncommon in the ferret as of this writing. There are anecdotal reports of hypothyroidism. Thyroiditis has been reported in ferrets with Aleutian disease.[82] Two cases of thyroid adenocarcinoma have also been reported.[82] Normal thyroid values can be found in chapter 8.

Gastrointestinal System

Numerous diseases affect the gastrointestinal (GI) tract in ferrets, often with similar clinical signs. The most common problems are covered here, but the differential diagnosis for gastrointestinal disorders should also include *Salmonella*, *Clostridia* sp. overgrowth, influenza, rotaviruses, Aleutian disease, lymphoma, mycobacteriosis, ingested toxins, and metabolic disease.[93]

Anal gland disease

Diseases of the anal glands are not commonly found in the United States because of the current practice of removing these glands in ferrets intended for the pet market.[94] The differential diagnosis for anal gland disorders includes infection, impaction, and neoplasia.

Infection of the anal sacculectomy sites can occur if any glandular tissue is left behind at the time of excision, leading to draining tracts in he perianal area (figure 24). Treatment includes appropriate antibiotics and surgical excision of the remaining tissue. (See chapter 6.)

One or both anal glands in ferrets can become impacted and/or infected. Signs of impaction include crying on defecation, decrease in diameter of stools ("ribbon-like"), excessive rubbing of the anal area on the floor, and obvious swelling. These glandular abscesses seldom burst and lancing is unnecessary.[94] Treatment involves a 7- to 10-day course of antibiotics and twice-daily hot compresses.[94] The gland is surgically removed when the swelling subsides. It is recommended that both glands be removed at the time of surgery to prevent further disease.[94] (See chapter 6.)

Dental disease

Deciduous teeth erupt at 14 days and continue appearing until the formula is complete: 2(I 4/3, C 1/1, Pm 3/3)= 30.[7] (I = incisor; C = canine; Pm = premolar; M = molar.) Permanent teeth start erupting between 50 and 74 days of age. The adult dental formula in ferrets is 2(I 3/3, C 1/1, Pm 3/3, M 1/2), a total of 34 teeth.[7]

Ferrets can develop plaque and tartar on their teeth. Bacterial buildup in the mouth can lead to endocarditis, cystitis, and kidney infections. Standard home dental care with a finger brush or a soft child's toothbrush and animal-approved toothpaste should be recommended to every new ferret owner.[95] Tartar can be inhibited by rubbing the teeth with Tartar Control Crest (Procter & Gamble, Cincinnati, OH) or Colgate (Colgate-Palmolive Co., New York, NY) several times weekly.[63] Dental prophylactic care with scaling and polishing of the teeth should be carried out as needed. Long-term periodontal disease can lead to tooth loss, gingivitis, and gum recession.

Ferrets are also prone to fracturing the tips of the canine teeth during rough play. If the pulp is exposed, either extract the affected tooth or perform a root canal to prevent abscessation.[95] Standard dental methods as used with cats are suitable for ferrets.

Tooth root abscesses of the molars and canine teeth have been reported in the ferret.[18] Clinical signs include facial swelling, pain on palpation of the sinuses or jaw, difficulty eating, dropping food, weight loss, and pawing at the site. Radiographs are recommended to determine the presence of bone lysis. Treat with antibiotics such as clindamycin (5.5–10 mg/kg PO every 12 hours) prophylactically before routine extraction under anesthesia.

Eosinophilic gastroenteritis

Eosinophilic gastroenteritis (EG) is a disease of unknown etiology involving invasion of the stomach, intestinal, and colonic mucosa with eosinophils. Eosinophilic invasion may also occur in the liver, spleen, and abdominal lymph nodes.[96] Dietary intolerance is suspected as a source of this disease in ferrets.[18] Affected patients are young to middle-aged and gender does not appear to be a factor.[96]

Clinical signs can include vomiting, diarrhea, anorexia, melena or hematochezia, lethargy, and weight loss.[96,97] Several cases have been seen with swollen erythematous footpads and ears.[94] Dry, crusted ears and generalized skin ulcerations have also been reported in two cases.[94] Enlarged mesenteric nodes and thickened loops of intestine may be palpable on physical examination.[96] The presumptive diagnosis of eosinophilic gastroenteritis is based on the combination of the preceding clinical signs with a peripheral eosinophilia (absolute eosinophilia of $1000 \times 10^3/\mu l$ or greater).[94,96] Note that not all cases of EG present with eosinophilia. Eosinophilic gastroenteritis should be differentiated from other causes of eosinophilia in the ferret, such as heartworm disease, parasites, or reactions to environmental allergens. Definite diagnosis requires an abdominal exploratory examination and biopsy of the small intestine and the mesenteric lymph nodes.[94,97] Treatment is usually based on potentially lifelong corticosteroids. Start with 0.1 mg/kg prednisone PO every 12 hours, and adjust the dosage upward as needed to control signs.[94] Signs usually resolve in 48 hours, but treatment should be continued for at least 4 weeks before attempt-g a reduction of the corticosteroid dosage. Signs frequently recur, nd corticosteroids are usually used for life. Hypoallergenic diets, uch as those used in cats, have been used with some success in these atients.[94] Raw turkey (both muscle and organ meat) or a feline ypoallergenic lamb and rice diet is recommended to reduce clinical igns and the amount of steroids needed for control of this disease.[94] he author (Brown) has successfully reduced the eosinophil count to ormal and caused remission of clinical signs in some cases with a ypoallergenic diet alone.

pizootic catarrhal enteritis

pizootic catarrhal enteritis (ECE) is a relatively new disease first oted in 1994 among ferrets in the show circuit on the East Coast of ie United States.[94,98] It causes necrosis of the mucosal epithelium ning the vilar tips, similar to parvovirus in the dog.[98] The actual rganism is unknown, but coronavirus- or rotavirus-type particles have een isolated from affected animals.[98,99] ECE is highly contagious, pread by the fecal–oral route, and can be carried on clothing and kin. Strict sanitation must be followed to prevent spread of this dis- ase to uninfected animals.[99] The incubation period is 2 to 3 days after xposure.[98] Severity of the disease depends on the age and condition f the host.

linical signs are nonspecific: vomiting (approximately 80% affected), thargy, and anorexia are seen early in the course of the disease.[98] iarrhea can range from mucus-laden green stools to the passing of rank blood.[98] In severely affected animals, profuse vomiting, bloody iarrhea, dehydration, and listlessness can lead to death within 8 hours.[99] All affected patients should be isolated with strict sanita- on protocols, similar to those used for parvovirus-infected dogs or ansmissible gastroenteritis-infected pigs.[29,99] The differential iagnosis includes rotavirus, proliferative colitis, ingested toxins, elicobacter gastritis, and eosinophilic gastroenteritis. The diagnosis made by ruling out other diseases because few affected animals can tolerate intestinal biopsy.[99] A detailed history including contact with other ferrets within 48 to 72 hours and outbreak in all ferrets in the household is very indicative of ECE. An elevated white blood cell (WBC) count may be seen, and a highly elevated SGPT on serum biochemistry is almost a hallmark of this disease.[100] Diagnostic blood work and fecal examination also reveal concurrent disease that might impede recovery of the patient.[99] This disease has a high morbidity (approaching 100%) but a low mortality (1–2%) with proper care.[98]

Treatment depends on the condition of the ferret. Those younger than 2 years may exhibit only a few days of green mucus-laden diarrhea and require only basic supportive care (oral or parenteral fluids, bland diet) as long as they are eating, drinking, and urinating normally. If anorexia develops, tempt the patient with poultry-based human baby food, a/d (Hill's Pet Products, Topeka, KS), or other liquid protein preparations. Treat mild dehydration with oral electrolyte solutions or subcutaneous lactated Ringer's solution (LRS). Loperamide (0.2 mg [1 cc]/kg PO every 12 hours) is an antidiarrheal drug that shortens the course of this disease in ferrets.[94] Kaolin-pectate (1–2 ml PO every 12–24 hours)[98] can be given to soothe potentially ulcerated areas of the digestive tract. Famotidine (0.25–0.5 mg/kg PO or IV every 24 hours) may resolve signs of nausea related to gastric pain.[98] If melena develops, add sucralfate (125 mg of liquid suspension PO every 6–8 hours). Antibiotics such as amoxicillin (10–25 mg/kg PO every 12 hours) are appropriate if secondary bacterial infections are suspected. Older ferrets, especially those with concurrent disease, require aggressive supportive care and regular monitoring for anemia caused by bleeding ulcers.[98] An incubator helps to maintain normothermia in debilitated animals, but be cautious of overheating.[99] Institute nutritional support, assist feeding if necessary. Hill's a/d (Hill's Pet Products, Topeka, KS) or liquid nutritional formula (Deliver 2.0, Mead Johnson Nutritionals, Evansville, IN) is recommended, warmed and syringe fed at 5 to 10 ml PO every 2 to 3 hours. Nonresponsive patients may benefit from steroids (prednisone 0.1–0.5 mg/kg every 12–24 hours).[94,99] Patients that are eating on their own can be discharged once the dehydration is corrected. Antibiotics should be continued for 2 weeks and anti-diarrheal agents used until stools are normal. Some older recovered ferrets with normal or slightly "grainy" stools have significant weight loss 3 weeks after the course of the initial disease. This may be a malabsorption problem caused by the severely damaged intestinal mucosa. Increasing the fat content of the diet seems to help, but dairy products should be avoided if diarrhea is present. Various combinations of blenderized beef liver, heavy cream, a/d (Hill's Pet Products, Topeka, KS), cooked egg, whipping cream, and strained-meat baby foods can be used to maintain weight.[94] Low doses of corticosteroids (prednisone 0.1–0.5 mg/kg every 12–24 hours) may aid in this situation.[98]

It is important to warn clients that recovered animals are carriers of ECE for 6 months or longer and should not be allowed contact with ferrets that have never been exposed. Disease can recur in patients that have been previously affected.[94]

Gastrointestinal foreign bodies

Foreign bodies in the GI tract are a common problem, especially in ferrets younger than 1 year of age. As mentioned in the husbandry section, ferrets have a tendency to chew and ingest latex, foam rubber, and occasionally cloth. After 1 year of age, this behavior greatly decreases. However, in the older animal, obstruction with trichobezoars becomes a more frequent problem (figure 18). It is recommended that owners offer a feline hairball laxative product regularly (see chapter 2).

Signs of GI foreign bodies vary greatly. In cases of gastric foreign bodies that are not causing acute obstructive disease, the signs can be vague and include any combination of the following: intermittent anorexia, abnormally thin stools ("pencil lead"), tarry stools, depression, gradual weight loss with eventual severe wasting, pawing at the mouth, and salivation. Vomiting does occur but is an infrequent finding with gastric foreign bodies. The ferret may become irritable and aggressive as a result of chronic pain. When a complete obstruction occurs, whether it is at the pylorus or in the small intestine, the signs are much more dramatic, as would be expected. The patient exhibits severe depression and dehydration, vomiting is more common, abdominal distention is seen (caused primarily by a gas-filled stomach), and death may occur in 24 to 48 hours. Seizures caused by severe electrolyte abnormalities in the end stages of obstruction are often mistaken for neurologic disease or toxin ingestion.

The different diagnoses for GI foreign bodies include EG, lymphoma or other neoplasia, gastric ulcers, gastric polyps, ECE, parasites, and proliferative bowel disease. The diagnosis is based primarily on the physical examination and radiography. The ferret abdomen is easily palpated, and foreign materials in the stomach or intestine are frequently identifiable. However, it may be difficult to palpate small trichobezoars, as they compress easily. The pet should be fasted for 4 to 6 hours before examination or radiography. Survey radiographs are used to reveal gastrointestinal tract obstruction. Radiographic signs of GI tract foreign body include a stomach grossly dilated with air and fluid, severe intestinal gas distention, or dense material evident in the stomach (figure 25). In ferrets, an air-distended stomach is an extreme emergency, and surgery cannot be avoided by merely decompressing the stomach. A barium series can be performed but is usually unnecessary. Exploratory laparotomy is recommended if clinical suspicion is high for a foreign body, despite negative diagnostic screening.

Exploratory surgery is the treatment of choice for GI foreign bodies. Ferrets are excellent surgical candidates, and the prognosis is good unless the animal was extremely debilitated before surgery. See chapter 6 for the surgical procedure.

Gastric ulcerative disease

Gastric and duodenal ulceration occurs most often in young ferrets (12–20 weeks) in stressful situations that include dietary changes, malnutrition, rapid growth, and concurrent disease.[101]

Research strongly suggests *Helicobacter mustelae* as the causative agent.[102] Nearly 100% of ferrets with clinical illness are naturally infected with this organism. Most ferrets are asymptomatic carriers of the bacteria. The signs of active disease in ferrets are anorexia, nausea, occasional vomiting, bruxism, melena, and wasting.[94,102] Severe cases present with dehydration and lethargy. Chronic gastric pain can cause behavioral changes and aggression.

The diagnosis is usually presumptive, based on clinical signs after ruling out other possibilities, such as GI neoplasia, GI foreign body, insulinoma, and toxin ingestion. Physical examination usually reveals weight loss and pain on cranial abdominal palpation. A CBC may indicate mild anemia and peripheral lymphocytosis.[94,102] Blood chemistry values are usually unremarkable. The diagnosis can be confirmed by biopsy or gastric wash, but it may be difficult to isolate the organism.[94,102] Histopathology reveals gastric or duodenal ulceration, lymphoplasmocytic gastritis, atrophy of the gastric mucosa, and achlorhydria.[94,102]

The treatment regimen is based on the severity of the clinical disease. Basic treatment includes antibiotics such as amoxicillin (10–25 mg/kg PO every 12 hours) and metronidazole (20 mg/kg PO every 12 hours), combined with bismuth subsalicylate (Pepto-Bismol original formula, Procter & Gamble, Cincinnati, OH; 17.5 mg/kg or 0.25 ml/kg PO every 4–6 hours).[102] There has been some controversy about the use in this disease of bismuth subsalicylate, which has been discontinued in human treatment protocols.[94] With severe clinical disease, supportive care with subcutaneous (SC) or intravenous fluids to correct dehydration is an essential part of the therapeutic regimen, which includes cimetidine (10 mg/kg every 8 hours PO, SC, or by slow IV bolus), sucralfate (1/8 of a 1-g tablet or 1.25 ml of the 100-mg/ml suspension PO every 6–8 hours), amoxicillin (20 mg/kg PO or SQ every 12 hours), and clarithromycin (Biaxin, Abbott Laboratories, Chicago, IL; 50 mg/kg PO every 24 hours). Treatment is for 14 days.[29] Proton pump inhibitors such as omeprazole (0.7 mg/kg PO every 12 hours) have been recommended to induce hypochlorhydria in the presence of ulcers.[102] In cases that are unresponsive to antibiotic therapy, low doses of corticosteroids control the disease and associated pain.[94] Prednisone (0.1–0.3 mg/kg PO every 12 hours) is recommended.[94] Chronic *Helicobacter mustelae* infections have been implicated in gastric neoplasia.[103,104]

Hepatic disease

Neoplasia, parasites, infectious agents, and toxin ingestion can cause hepatic disease in the ferret. Hepatic lipidosis can be seen with severe anorexia and wasting. The most common neoplasm is metastatic, usually from an insulinoma, but can include lymphoma, hemagiosarcoma, hemangioma, and tumors arising from hepatocyte and biliary tissues.[60]

Hepatic disease has no age or gender predilection. Clinical signs include vomiting, lethargy, inappetence, diarrhea with or without melena, and icterus. In chronic disease, the most significant finding is chronic diarrhea and gradual wasting. A fecal smear and flotation are used to screen for parasites. The CBC is usually normal, although the WBC count can be elevated with a left shift in severe, acute infections.[105] Blood chemistry evaluation of liver enzyme values shows an increase in alanine aminotransferase (ALT), serum alkaline phosphatase (SAP), and total bilirubin concentration.[105] In ferrets, ALT is most concentrated in the liver.[105] Ultrasonography is very useful in diagnosing hepatic lesions. Ultrasound-guided biopsy or abdominal endoscopy or exploratory examination with a biopsy of the liver will determine a definitive diagnosis.

Treatment is based on the diagnosis. Secondary hepatic lipidosis is treated with supportive care and correction of the underlying primary disease. Antibiotics such as enrofloxacin (5–10 mg/kg PO every 12 hours) or amoxicillin (20 mg/kg PO every 12 hours) in combination with metronidazole (20 mg/kg PO every 12 hours) are recommended. Additional therapy can include lactulose syrup (0.1 cc/kg [10 g/15 ml] PO every 12 hours), fluid therapy, vitamin B complex (0.25 cc/kg IM initially, then orally at the feline dose), and vitamin K (0.15–1.0 cc/kg IM). Frequent high-quality meals encourage weight gain. There have been two reported cases of biliary coccidiosis in a ferret, but no treatment is mentioned.[29,106] Supportive care is recommended in cases of suspected toxin ingestion or infectious disease. Hepatic abscesses can require surgical excision or marsupialization to the abdominal wall. Focal hepatic neoplasia can be surgically excised. Treatment of generalized hepatic neoplasia or metastasis has not been successful.

Megaesophagus

Acquired megaesophagus has been reported in ferrets.[107,108] The etiology is unknown at this time.[107] The presenting complaints are regurgitation and weight loss. Clinical signs include difficulty swallowing, lethargy, inappetence, coughing, and choking.[107,108] Physical examination reveals cachexia, dehydration, weakness, ptyalism, bruxism, crackles on auscultation, and/or crepitus in the cervical region.[107,108] The differential diagnosis includes esophageal or gastric foreign body, gastritis, and respiratory disease.[108] Diagnosis is by radiography or endoscopy. Concurrent malnutrition, hepatic lipidosis, and/or aspiration pneumonia are usually found. Although supportive care according to canine protocols (i.e., feeding meals in an elevated position) can be attempted, the prognosis is poor.[107,108]

Neoplasia

Several types of neoplasia occur in the GI tract. Squamous cell carcinoma has been reported in the oral cavity in seven ferrets.[103] These tumors vary in appearance. Clinical signs are usually related to changes in prehension and/or chewing.[60,103] The differential diagnoses for oral masses also includes fibrosarcoma[60] (figure 26). This appears as a firm, smooth oral mass that grows rapidly.[60] Treatment of these tumors, including aggressive surgical removal and chemotherapy, has not been rewarding.[60,103] The prognosis is poor.

There have been several reports of pyloric adenocarcinoma, causing gastric distention, vomiting, anorexia, dehydration, and lethargy.[104,109]

The differential diagnosis includes peritoneal mesothelioma, lymphoma, and GI foreign bodies.[60,110] *Helicobacter mustelae* infection may be implicated in gastric neoplasia.[103,104] Diagnosis is by biopsy and the prognosis is poor. Chemotherapy for GI neoplasia has been unrewarding.

Other reported GI tract neoplasms include salivary gland adenocarcinoma, leiomyoma and leiomyosarcomas of the intestinal tract, and squamous cell carcinoma of the anus.[59] Hepatic neoplasia is covered under Hepatic Disease.

Parasites

Gastrointestinal parasites seldom cause clinical disease in ferrets. However, a fecal flotation and smear for parasites (especially protozoans) should be included in any diagnostic workup for GI disease. The most common intestinal parasites reported in ferrets are *Cryptosporidium*, coccidia, and *Giardia*.[108]

Coccidiosis causes diarrhea, weight loss, dehydration, and lethargy.[111] Diagnosis is based on fecal examination. Treatment is sulfadimethoxine (30 mg/kg PO every 24 hours) or trimethoprim-sulfadiazine oral suspension (30 mg/kg PO every 24 hours) for 14 days.[112] A fecal flotation should be performed 1 week after treatment ends.[112]

Cryptosporidium infection is not treatable. Clinical signs include anorexia, depression, and yellowish diarrhea. Oocysts are found on fecal analysis. The disease is usually subclinical, either self-limiting or rapidly fatal when triggered by stress or dexamethasone exposure.[113] Owners should be warned of the zoonotic potential of *Cryptosporidium* in immunocompromised individuals.[114] Prevention and control are the best methods of avoiding this infection.[111] Perform fecal examinations on any new ferrets brought into a household and quarantine them separately for at least 2 weeks before introduction to the rest of the group. Appropriate sanitation will remove fecal material before sporulation of oocysts can occur.[111]

Giardia is commonly found on fecal smears in healthy animals, existing as a subclinical infection. Clinically ill animals exhibit soft, grainy stools and weight loss. The recommended treatment is metronidazole (35 mg/kg PO every 12–24 hours) for 14 days.[94] A fecal smear should be reexamined 1 week after the end of treatment. Giardia is spread by fecal–oral contact and has zoonotic potential. Clients should be encouraged to use proper sanitation when handling ill ferrets. Giardia outbreaks are difficult to eradicate, especially in colonies.

Proliferative bowel disease

Proliferative bowel disease (PBD) is an uncommon cause of GI tract disease in a pet ferret. It is caused by an intracellular Desulfovibrio sp. and may include coinfection with coccidia.[115] This disease is usually seen in animals younger than 14 months of age.[97,116] The pathogenesis is not completely understood, but environmental stresses probably interact with infectious agents.[115] The disease most commonly affects the colon but may also be present in the small bowel.[116]

PBD can present as either an acute or chronic disease. Clinical signs include severe weight loss, inappetence, and lethargy, with the most prominent sign being frequent, painful passing of mucus-coated or blood-streaked stools.[97,117] Rectal prolapse is a common sequela.[93] Some patients exhibit central nervous system (CNS) signs such as ataxia, head tilts, and muscle tremors.[97,116] A presumptive diagnosis of PBD is based on these clinical signs, particularly the painful defecation. Physical examination reveals a thickened colon or small intestine, as well as enlarged mesenteric lymph nodes on abdominal palpation. This is often enough information to initiate treatment in the acutely ill animal. A definitive diagnosis is based on intestinal mucosal biopsy, which can be accomplished via abdominal exploratory examination or endoscopy. Histopathology reveals hyperplastic mucosa, and silver stain demonstrates the organism within the epithelium.[116]

PBD is treated with chloramphenicol (50 mg/kg PO, SC, or IM every

12 hours) for 14 to 21 days.[97,116] Recurrence may require a second round of treatment. Hillyer has had success using metronidazole (20 mg/kg PO every 12 hours) for the same period of time.[97] Alternative treatments include tylosin (10 mg/kg PO every 12 hours) or sulfasalazine (10–15 mg/kg PO every 6–8 hours). Use other supportive care as needed. Rectal prolapses normally resolve with treatment but may require a purse-string suture if they persist.[93]

Salivary mucocele

Several cases of salivary gland mucocele have been seen in the ferret.[64,118] Clinical signs include a soft, fluctuant swelling over the face and head. Aspiration of the mass reveals saliva. Surgical removal is usually curative. It may be difficult to find the ruptured duct, leading to recurrence. Marsupialization of the gland may be necessary in these cases.

Integument

Ferrets normally shed twice yearly, in the spring and fall. Coat patterns and color can change significantly after shedding.[6] Intact animals often show even more marked coat color and texture changes than neutered ferrets. Although molting usually takes place gradually, it can also be a very dramatic change, with the entire undercoat lost in 1 to 2 days.[6] The winter coat is thicker and sometimes longer than the summer coat. Hair regrowth can be very slow in the nonmolting season, and the hair may not grow back until the next seasonal shedding period if lost with clipping or shaving.[6] Hair regrowth may be preceded by blue discoloration of the skin; this is a normal occurrence, caused by new hairs within the dermis.

Alopecia

The most common cause of generalized bilaterally symmetrical alopecia in the intact female is the prolonged estrous cycle (see Urogenital System later in this chapter) (figure 27). Ovarian remnants left during

ovariohysterectomy (OVH) produce the same signs in a spayed
female. Signs usually occur within 8 to 10 months of the OVH. An
ovariohysterectomy or ovarian remnant removal via exploratory
surgery (see chapter 6) is the treatment of choice. A CBC and platelet
count should be obtained before surgery to determine the presence of
bone marrow suppression. When the haircoat regrows it may be a different shade, length, and texture and the mask pattern may change.
(See Urogenital System for more information.)

In ferrets 2 years of age or older, the most common cause of bilaterally symmetrical alopecia is adrenal-associated endocrinopathy
(figure 22). Pruritus, dry skin, and changes in the texture of the skin
can also occur. The differential diagnosis includes ovarian remnants
and reproductive neoplasia. (See the Endocrine and Reproduction
sections for more detail.)

Alopecia of the tail occurs in both intact and neutered animals of any
age and either sex (figure 28). The etiology is unknown, but the condition is likely to be endocrine in origin because of its seasonal
occurrence. It coincides with the fall shedding period, when the length
of daylight hours is shortened, so photoperiod may have some effect
as well.[6] Some ferrets repeat this cycle of tail hair loss every year, and
other individuals are presented with this condition sporadically. It is
important to note that if the hair loss is persistent throughout the year
or if it progresses above the base of the tail, adrenal disease should be
considered. Clinical signs include a gradual loss of hair from the tip of
the tail and extending cranially. The hair may be sparse or totally gone
from the tail base to the tip. There may also be a reddish brown, waxy
deposit or comedones on the skin of the tail. The condition usually
resolves in 1 to 3 months without therapy. Treatment entails daily
washing of the affected area with antibacterial shampoo or a benzoyl
peroxide preparation.

Poor nutrition, particularly a diet that is deficient in high-quality animal protein and/or fat, can result in a dry, sparse coat that epilates
easily and may even have small patches of alopecia. Correcting the

diet should result in an improved coat in 1 to 2 months. Ferrets kept in temperatures over 80°F or in conditions of low humidity may also develop a sparse and dry coat. Cooling down the environment and adding fatty acid supplements to the diet should improve the coat condition in 2 to 4 weeks. Exposure to clay-based cat litters can also cause a brittle haircoat.

Fungal infection

Dermatophytosis is uncommon in ferrets. Ferrets are susceptible to infection by either *Microsporum canis* or *Trichophyton mentagrophytes*, most often by contact with a feline carrier or its bedding.[6,119] Clinical signs include papules that spread into the classic circular areas of alopecia, with or without pruritus, and thickened hyperkeratotic skin. Ferrets are probably not carriers and usually heal spontaneously. If necessary, shave local lesions and treat topically with antifungal medications, keratolytic shampoos, or povidone scrubs. In refractory cases, use griseofulvin (25 mg/kg PO every 24 hours) for 21 to 30 days. Warn owners of the zoonotic potential of fungal disease, treat other household pets, and encourage strict sanitation of the environment.

Other fungal dermatopathies are rare in the ferret. Several cases of *Actinomyces* infection have been noted.[29] Systemic *Aspergillus* has been seen.[18] Fungi should be ruled out when diagnosing draining tracts or persistent unresponsive dermatitis.

Infectious dermatopathies

Ferrets in the United States rarely present with bacterial skin disease. Abscesses are most commonly associated with puncture wounds. Clinical signs of bacterial dermatitis include hyperkeratosis, alopecia, and excoriations. Use skin scrapings to rule out ectoparasites. The exudate should be Gram stained and culture and sensitivity testing of the lesion used to determine the organisms involved.[119] Skin biopsies are recommended when cytology is inconclusive. The differential diagnois for bacterial skin infection includes cutaneous neoplasia, distemper, eosinophilic gastroenteritis, fungal infection, ectoparasites, and endocrine disorders. *Staphylococcus* sp., *Streptococcus* sp., *Corynebacterium*, *Pasteurella*, and *Actinomyces* have been isolated from ferret skin infections.[119] Treat with topical antibacterial shampoos and systemic antibiotics on the basis of culture results.

The anal glands can become abscessed. Surgical excision is the treatment of choice (see chapter 6). Treat with antibiotics before surgery to decrease swelling.

The distemper virus produces skin lesions in the course of disease, but these are very specific and easy to differentiate from other disorders (figure 28) and include hyperemia and crusting of the lips, chin, eyelids, and inguinal and perineal area and hyperkeratosis of the footpads (see Multisystemic Diseases).[119]

Cutaneous neoplasia

The skin is the third most common site of neoplasia in the ferret.[59] In the United States, cutaneous neoplasms account for the majority of skin masses on ferrets. Because the potential exists for metastasis with some types of cutaneous neoplasm, the recommended treatment is immediate surgical excision.[60] Chest radiographs are recommended before surgery to rule out metastasis. Fortunately, the majority of these proliferative lesions are slow growing, and removal is often curative. Electrosurgery should be used for quick excision of small skin masses. Histopathology is recommended to determine the prognosis and possible use of chemotherapy or radiation therapy.

The most common skin tumor in ferrets is basal cell in origin.[59] These have been seen in ferrets older than 2 years, with a predilection for females.[59] The appearance varies from pedunculated to plaquelike, wartlike, or cystic, and the tumors may be ulcerated.[59,119] Wide surgical excision is curative. Radiation therapy is recommended for invasive or nonoperable tumors.[120]

Another common neoplasm in the ferret is the cutaneous mastocytoma or mast cell tumor.[60,121] It usually occurs in ferrets 3 years of age and older. Mast cell tumors have a very specific appearance as a hairless, round, raised "button-like" lesion, which may be smooth or have a crusted surface due to pruritic irritation (figure 29). Mast cell tumors can range in size from a millimeter to over a centimeter. The size can fluctuate over time. Mast cell tumors can also present as diffuse lesions that can be several centimeters in diameter and may be confused with a more generalized dermatitis. A biopsy is necessary for a definitive diagnosis. Patchy areas of alopecia (not bilaterally symmetrical) may occur on the body, and these resolve when the mast cell tumor is removed. Mast cell tumors can occur on any part of the body and may be found singly or in groups of two or more. Treatment is complete surgical excision. Recurrence is rare at the site of removal, but they may occur on or in other areas of the body.

Sebaceous gland adenomas and adenocarcinomas occur in ferrets of any age.[60,103,122] They appear as a raised cauliflower-type lesion, a raised ulcerated lesion, or as a bluish lump under the skin anywhere on the body (figure 30). Males may develop these tumors around the prepuce, where they probably arise from the preputial glands.[60,121] Females develop sebaceous gland adenomas around the vulva. Adenocarcinomas grow rapidly in size and may aggressively metastasize to other organs. Adenomas, as would be expected, grow more slowly and remain only locally invasive. Expedient and complete surgical removal of these neoplasms is essential. In cases of preputial gland neoplasm, excise and biopsy at least one inguinal lymph node at the time of surgery to determine whether the disease has metastasized. The prognosis must be guarded in cases of sebaceous gland adenocarcinoma; however, consultation with an oncologist and use of radiation and/or chemotherapy may be helpful in some cases.[60]

Squamous cell carcinomas also occur in the ferret.[60,103,123] They

appear as a nodule with an ulcerated surface, but they may also
be disseminated.[123] Complete and expedient surgical excision is the
treatment of choice because of the possibility of metastasis.

Fibromas and fibrosarcomas occur on the extremities and in the
mouth.[60] They present as well-circumscribed dermal or subcutaneous
masses.[60,121] Radiographs of the affected area should be obtained to
determine bone involvement. If possible, remove the tumor and
affected bone. Metastasis has been reported.[18] Fibromas and fibrosarcomas may also occur internally at a variety of sites.

Lymphoma, although a common neoplastic disease in ferrets, is occasionally seen as a skin lesion.[60,121,124] There are several reported cases
of lymphoma associated with the prepuce.[60,121,124] With early and
complete excision there is a fair prognosis against recurrence.
Chemotherapy was used in a case of cutaneous epitheliotropic lymphoma in conjunction with antibiotics and regular soothing shampoos
with some success.[126] (See Multisystemic Diseases—Lymphoma for
more information.)

Other cutaneous neoplasias including sebaceous epitheliomas, rhab-
domyosarcoma, myxosarcoma of the subcutis, myelosarcoma,
leiomyosarcoma, papillary cystadenoma, hemangioma, hemangiosarcoma, histiocytoma, neurofibroma, and neurilemmoma have been seen
in the ferret.[59,60,72,103,119] Considering the ferret's propensity for developing neoplasia in general, anything would appear possible!

Ectoparasites

A common external parasite in the ferret is the flea, *Ctenocephalides
felis*.[6,119] Ferrets are natural hosts for the flea but appear to be fairly
tolerant and only occasionally develop skin lesions as a result. Heavy
infestation can lead to anemia and lethargy, as well as pruritus and
alopecia of the dorsum of the neck.[119] No flea products are currently
approved by the U.S. Department of Agriculture (USDA) for use in
ferrets. If only a few fleas are present, bathe thoroughly and comb

daily with a flea comb to remove the parasite, and treat the environment simultaneously. Generally, flea products that are approved for use in cats will be safe in ferrets.[6] Toxicity can occur if flea products are groomed off the skin and coat and ingested, in which case the ferret should be treated with standard antidotes for the product involved. Flea collars should never be used, as they are easily removed and eaten by the pet.[6] New flea products, such as imidacloprid (Advantage, Bayer Corporation, Shawnee Mission, KS), lufenuron (Program, Ciba Animal Health, Ciba-Geigy Corporation, Greensboro, NC), and fipronil (Frontline, Rhone-Merieux Inc., Athens, GA), have proven effective as once-monthly treatments for fleas in dogs and cats. Anecdotal use of imidacloprid, using 0.1 ml of the lowest available cat dose placed at the base of the skull, has been effective in controlling a flea infestation in a shelter situation when applied monthly. Lufenuron is an oral medication that produces sterility in fleas that have been exposed to the drug through a blood meal. The pill form is difficult to administer to ferrets, and the dosage is unknown. Because of the small size of ferrets, use of this medication is not recommended because the fleas must bite the animal for exposure. According to the staff at Rhone-Merieux, there have been no reported problems with fipronil in ferrets.[127] The recommended dosage is half the package of feline topical, applied high on the neck.[127]

Ear mites (*Otodectes cyanotis*) are common in ferrets and may be found incidentally on physical examination. Normal earwax in the ferret is dark brown and heavy in comparison to that in other species. Microscopic examination of the exudate is recommended annually to detect the presence of mites. The recommended treatment involves thorough cleansing of the ear canals and topical application of ivermectin (Ivomec, Merck, Whitehouse Station, NJ), diluted with propylene glycol and placed in each ear (0.5–1.0 mg/kg divided in both ears). Repeat the treatment in 2 weeks.[6] Miticide preparations approved for use in cats can also be used for treatment, but daily administration decreases owner compliance. All animals in the house-

old should be treated, and living areas should be treated and/or
washed as appropriate. Recurrent infestations can be caused by
improper cleansing of the ear canals before medicating, small ear
canals, mites present on other areas of the body, lack of client compliance, or reinfestation by other pets or the environment. Recommended
treatment includes the topical ear medication regimen combined with
bathing or administering topical antiparasitic preparations to the entire
animal weekly until it is mite free.[119]

Ticks may be found on ferrets allowed to go outdoors or abandoned in
a wooded area. Remove ticks carefully with forceps or hemostats to
prevent human exposure to disease. There is no documented evidence
that tick-borne diseases affect ferrets.

Infestation with *Sarcoptes* sp. is uncommon in the ferret. Transmission
is usually via an infected household pet through either direct contact
or exposure to infested bedding.[119] Clinical signs of localized infection
include crusting of the feet with erythema, hyperemia, and intense
pruritus.[6,119] The nails may become deformed or slough.[119] The clinical signs of generalized disease include focal alopecia, scaling, and
pruritus, but this is rare.[6,119] Diagnosis is based on clinical signs and
response to treatment. Skin scrapings are seldom diagnostic; therefore,
biopsies are used if a definitive diagnosis is required. Treat with ivermectin (0.2–0.4 mg/kg SC) and repeat every 14 days until clinical
signs have resolved.[6,119] Soak the feet daily with warm water, gently
debride softened crusts, and trim diseased claws.[119] Treat all animals
in the household, and advise thorough cleaning of the environment to
prevent reinfection. Warn the owner of the zoonotic potential of this
parasite.

Cutaneous myiasis has been noted in the ferret.[119,128] Flesh fly
(*Wohlfahrtia vigil*) infestation is seen in ferrets maintained or abandoned outdoors, causing irritation to the face, neck, and flanks.[128]
Cuterebra larvae can cause subdermal cysts.[128] Treatment for myiasis
involves careful removal of the larvae intact, to avoid leaving a source

of infection or precipitating an anaphylactic response.[119] Debride the wound(s) and apply topical and/or systemic antibiotics as appropriate.[119] Provide supportive care for secondary sepsis or shock.[119]

Multisystemic Diseases

Aleutian disease virus

Aleutian disease virus (ADV) is a parvovirus that was discovered originally in mink (*Mustela vison*).[97,129,130] The ferret strain of this disease is an apparently weaker mutation of the mink parvovirus.[130] In ferrets ADV is manifest as an immune-mediated disease resulting in lymphocytic infiltration of multiple organs, particularly the meninges of the brain.[131] It is transmitted horizontally by fecal/urine to oral contact and fomites and vertically from dam to kits.[132] Most adult ferrets exposed to the virus do not develop disease. Some animals become asymptomatic carriers for months to years. Some of these carriers may revert to a negative state (based on an immunofluorescent antibody test) at any time. Clinical signs vary in ferrets that develop the active form of ADV. The most common sign is a progressive posterior weakness and ataxia that eventually ends in complete paralysis accompanied by wasting, splenomegaly, hepatomegaly, lethargy, pallor, and melena.[129,130] The disease may be acute or chronic with signs progressing over several weeks to months.[133] Chronic disease can lead to glomerulonephritis and eventual renal failure. Another reported presentation is that of a sudden change in personality, with the pet becoming extremely hyperactive followed by lethargy, anorexia, and death in a few days. Histopathologically, these animals had lymphocytic infiltration of the thyroid gland, which may have led initially to a stimulation of the thyroid with resultant temporary hyperthyroidism.[18]

The differential diagnosis includes gastric ulcers, eosinophilic gastroenteritis, neoplasia, cardiomyopathy, rabies, CNS disease, insulinoma, metabolic disease, environmental toxicity, and estrogen-induced anemia.[132]

Diagnosis is based on clinical signs and a positive immunofluorescent antibody (IFA) test for antibodies to the ADV antigen or counterelectrophoresis proof of infection. A number of laboratories across the country can perform these tests. Specific titers can also be determined. The possibility of false negatives does exist. Diagnostic testing often reveals lymphocytosis (but this is also seen with lymphoma, which is a more common disease) and hypergammaglobulinemia.[129,130,133]

It should be noted that many clinically normal ferrets might have positive Aleutian IFA tests. These animals may be carriers, but they may never develop clinical signs. The author (Brown) tested over 500 ferrets at a local ferret shelter and found 13% to have positive titers to Aleutian disease on fluorescent antibody test, with only 2 of those animals developing clinical disease over a 3-year period. Therefore, it is not recommended that healthy animals that test positively be euthanized. It is also unnecessary to remove positive animals from a household where all animals have already been exposed. However, in the breeding facility, it would not be wise to use positive animals as breeders or to expose them to neonates. Breeding facilities should test all animals before they are introduced, quarantine them for 1 month, and then test again. If they are negative the second time, they may enter the colony.

There is no successful treatment for Aleutian disease. Supportive care increases the quality of life and improves clinical signs for a varying period of time.[132] Corticosteroid therapy may cause temporary remission of signs, but it is not curative and may worsen renal lesions.

Canine distemper virus

Early canine distemper is often confused with an upper respiratory or eye infection.[134] The incubation period is 7 to 21 days, and the initial sign is a unilateral or bilateral, serous, ocular discharge that quickly becomes purulent. Conjunctivitis, often with blepharospasm and photophobia, develops.[135] The conjunctivitis is unresponsive to treatment, and the patient becomes lethargic and depressed and gradually loses its appetite. Coughing, vomiting, and diarrhea follow. Within 24 to 72 hours of the onset of signs, erythema followed by crusting of the integument appears on the lips, chin, around the nares, around the anus, and in the inguinal area[135] (figure 31). The footpads become hyperkeratotic.[135] In some patients there may be a neurotropic episode before death. CNS signs include torticollis, incoordination, nystagmus, blindness, and seizures. The patient may live for several days to more than a week, but the disease is 99% fatal. A presumptive diagnosis can be made on the basis of a history of exposure and the presence of the mentioned dermatologic clinical signs (rash and swelling), as these are pathognomonic for canine distemper virus (CDV). For a more definitive diagnosis, perform a fluorescent antibody test on a conjunctival scraping, mucous membrane scraping, peripheral blood smear, or buffy coat.[130] Because of the severity of this disease, euthanasia is strongly recommended for all affected ferrets. One ferret that tested positive for CDV had a prolonged life span with supportive care.[136] Recommended treatment in cases of mild distemper includes systemic broad-spectrum antibiotics to treat secondary bacterial infections, antimicrobial ophthalmic ointment, fluid therapy, nebulization, and hypoallergenic shampoo for skin irritation.[136] Although treatment is not available to cure CDV, supportive care can increase the quality of life until CNS signs appear.

Another less common syndrome of canine distemper, seen by the author (Brown) and reported to her by a breeder with a confirmed distemper outbreak, is one in which the ferret goes directly into a neurotropic episode with no other signs. The patient may be presented in status epilepticus or suddenly may become extremely aggressive. An insulinoma is the most frequent cause of seizures in the ferret but is easily diagnosed by demonstrating a low blood glucose level or response to oral or IV glucose. It is extremely difficult to diagnose distemper in this form, and rabies has to be considered in the differential diagnosis. If anyone is bitten by an animal being presented in this manner (and excluding the possibility of insulinoma), it would be best

o euthanize the patient and have a rabies examination performed on
the brain tissue.

Prevention of CDV is by proper vaccination with an approved vaccine.
(See chapter 3, Preventative Health Program.)

Lymphoma

Lymphoma is a common neoplasm in ferrets.[59] It is speculated that
this particular neoplasia, like the viral leukemia diseases of the cat, is
caused by an oncogenic retrovirus.[137] Lymphoma can affect ferrets at
any age and of either sex. There are currently two recognized forms of
this disease in ferrets: a rapidly progressive form in ferrets younger
than 1 year of age and a slowly progressive form in older ferrets.[138]
The rapidly progressive form is manifest as a peripheral
lymphadenopathy, with an anterior mediastinal mass(es) or
lymphoblastic leukemia and sudden death.[138] The prognosis is poor,
with survival usually less than 2 months after diagnosis if not
treated.[138] Many ferrets with the slowly progressive form are totally
asymptomatic for months to years.[138,139] Lymphoma should always be
considered a systemic disease, even in cases with the outward appearance of being localized. Signs of lymphoma are variable, depending
on the organs affected. Clinical signs can include anorexia, lethargy,
weight loss, splenomegaly, localized lymph node enlargement, mediastinal or sternal lymph node enlargement with accompanying
dyspnea, wasting, frequently recurring upper respiratory infections,
recurring fevers, and general lethargy.[60,139,140] The patient may
demonstrate a persistently high WBC count (over 10,000 x 10^3/μl)
with an absolute lymphocyte count over 3500 x 10^3/μl or a lower total
WBC count with lymphocytes persisting at 60% or higher.[138,141] Note
that ferrets younger than 6 months can have a naturally occurring lymphocytosis, as can older ferrets with chronic infection, which can lead
to a mistaken presumptive diagnosis of lymphoma.[140] Rarely, atypical
lymphocytes are present in the WBC count analysis.[140] Anemia is also
a common finding.[140]

Lymphoma is the presumptive diagnosis based on these clinical signs, the CBC count values, and radiographic or ultrasound evidence of internal masses. A definitive diagnosis is reached via cytology, biopsy, or fluid analysis. In thoracic disease, evaluate the cytology of any effusions present. A fine-needle aspirate of large masses can be diagnostic. Needle aspirates of peripheral lymph nodes are seldom successful because of the small size of the node and the large perinodal fat pad. In cases of persistent lymphocytosis (even if the animal is clinically normal) or peripheral lymphadenopathy, a lymph nodectomy should be performed (see chapter 4, Tissue Biopsies). The popliteal lymph node is easily accessible. Lymph nodectomy provides a more definitive diagnosis than a bone marrow aspirate.[60] Avoid the use of the gastric lymph node for diagnosis, as it is often enlarged in ferrets with subclinical gastritis.[60] Bone marrow aspirates can be taken from the femur (see chapter 4). Splenic aspirates may also be performed in ferrets with significant splenomegaly (see chapter 4), but they are frequently nondiagnostic.

In ferrets older than 6 months that are clinically normal, yet exhibit peripheral lymphocytosis, repeat the WBC count in 3 to 4 weeks to see whether the trend is persistent.[60] If the lymphocytosis persists, perform a popliteal lymph nodectomy and histopathology. If the lymph node is hyperplastic on microscopic exam, check a CBC count at 6-month intervals and repeat the lymph node removal in 1 year if the lymphocytosis trend persists. Some cases of lymphoid hyperplasia develop into malignant lymphoma at a later date. Also consider testing for Aleutian disease, because this can also present with lymphocytosis.

Lymphoma can be treated with chemotherapy.[60,142,143] Ferrets in general are resilient chemotherapy patients with a high tolerance level for the drugs used.[60] Although the prognosis is guarded in all cases of lymphoma, in some ferrets chemotherapy can result in remission of the disease for months to years.[60] Ferrets should be thoroughly evaluated before chemotherapy, including a CBC count, serum biochemistry screen, radiographs to track the progress of thoracic disease, and a bone marrow aspirate. Chemotherapy is not recommended more than 50% of the bone marrow consists of neoplastic cells. It may benefit the patient to remove the spleen prior to therapy if it is grossly enlarged or shows evidence of lymphoma on an aspirate.

Candidates for chemotherapy should be selected carefully. Ferrets that have received corticosteroids for concurrent disease conditions (e.g., insulinoma) may be refractory to chemotherapy. Asymptomatic but clinically diagnosed lymphoma patients should not be treated but should be monitored as outlined above. The author (Brown) has seen the best response in ferrets that have the disease in the mediastinum, spleen, skin, or peripheral lymph nodes; do not have concurrent systemic disease; have more than 50% normal WBCs in the bone marrow; and are in good physical condition.[60] Ferrets that respond poorly or not at all to chemotherapy are those that have multifocal disease, or infiltration of the liver, intestines, abdomen, solitary lymph nodes, and/or bone marrow with 50% or more neoplastic cell populations.[60]

Asymptomatic ferrets may live relatively normal lives for 1 to 3 years before they become clinically ill.[60] It is particularly important not to prescribe corticosteroids alone for a patient if chemotherapy is ever to be considered in the future. The use of corticosteroids prior to institution of other chemotherapeutic agents may lead to drug resistance and failure of therapy.

Numerous chemotherapy protocols have been described for lymphoma in many species. Modifications can be made for ferrets. Consultation with a veterinary oncologist and use of a cancer therapy text are also advised.[60] Of course, proper safety guidelines must be followed to protect staff and clients whenever chemotherapeutic agents are used.

The author (Brown) has had varying success with a number of different chemotherapy protocols over the years. The current one used was presented by Dr. Karen Rosenthal in Veterinary Clinics of North America Exotic Pet Medicine II, January 1994. This protocol has been well tolerated by properly screened ferret patients.

WEEK	DRUG	DOSE
1	Vincristine	0.07 mg/kg IV
	Asparaginase	400 IU/kg IP
2	Cytoxan	10 mg/kg SC
3	Doxorubicin	1 mg/kg IV
4	Vincristine	0.07 mg/kg IV
5	Cytoxan	10 mg/kg SC
6	Doxorubicin	1 mg/kg IV
7	No treatment	
8	Vincristine	0.07 mg/kg IV
9	No treatment	
10	Cytoxan	10 mg/kg SC
11	No treatment	
12	Vincristine	0.07 mg/kg IV
13	No treatment	
14	Methotrexate	0.5 mg/kg IV
15	No treatment	
16*	Vincristine	0.07 mg/kg IV
17	No treatment	
18	Cytoxan	10 mg/kg SC
19	No treatment	
20	Doxorubicin	1 mg/kg IV
21	No treatment	
22	Vincristine	0.07 mg/kg IV
23	No treatment	
24	Cytoxan	10 mg/kg SC

25	No treatment	
26	Vincristine	0.07 mg/kg IV
27	No treatment	
28**	Methotrexate	0.5 mg/kg IV

After week 28 the chemotherapy may be stopped or continued in sequence (from * to **) biweekly, or any variation up to therapy once monthly in sequence may be used. Therapy is considered successful if organomegaly or masses are resolved, peripheral lymphocytes are 40% or lower, or the absolute lymphocyte count is less than 3000 x 10^3/μl for at least 3 months.[18,144]

The patient should be started with prednisone (0.5 mg/kg PO every 12 hours) on the first day of therapy. At presentation, the patient should be weighed and blood drawn for a CBC count (avoid the cephalic vein) before chemotherapy for that day begins. The patient should be provided with water but no food. If the WBC count is over 2000 x 10^3/μl, the PCV is greater than 30%, and the ferret is in good clinical condition, proceed with chemotherapy as determined for that day. If the WBC count is between 1000 and 2000 x 10^3/μl, administer filgrastim (a human granulocyte colony-stimulating factor) and determine fitness for chemotherapy based on physical examination. If the WBC count is below 1000 x 10^3/μl, postpone chemotherapy and administer filgrastim and necessary supportive care. Recheck the CBC count in 3 to 4 days. Do not proceed with chemotherapy unless the WBC count is greater than 2000 x 10^3/μl. If the PCV falls below 25%, administer erythropoietin and discontinue chemotherapy until the PCV is greater than 30%. Complete other diagnostic tests such as serum biochemistries and radiographs as needed on the basis of clinical signs.[18]

Use isoflurane anesthesia without premedication for all IV administration of chemotherapy agents. Place a 23- to 24-g butterfly catheter in the cephalic vein. Flush the catheter with a minimum of 3 cc of saline before chemotherapy. Dilute the chemotherapeutic agent in 5 cc of nonheparinized saline. Administer the chemotherapy drug slowly, and then flush the catheter with 3 cc of saline. If IV chemotherapeutic agents are injected outside the vein, flood the area with saline, use local dexamethasone, apply cold packs, and bandage the leg. Offer food and water when the patient is ambulatory. Discharge the patient when recovery is complete.

It is common for chemotherapy patients to lose weight in the third or fourth week of treatment. The diet should be supplemented with additional feeding, by syringe if necessary. Hill's a/d (Hill's Pet Products, Topeka, KS) or meat baby food can be mixed with Deliver 2.0 (Mead-Johnson, Evansville, IN), heavy cream, goat's milk, or blenderized beef liver to provide additional fat and protein to the diet. Feed 20 cc/kg up to four times daily. Additional supportive nutritional supplements include vitamin C, Pau d'Arco, pycnogenol, and echinacea. Vitamin C (25–50 mg/kg PO twice a day) is used in the buffered, ester, or chelated form as it causes less GI upset.[60] Start at 100 mg every 12 hours and gradually work up to the highest dose (over several weeks) that does not cause soft stools. Mixing powder from capsules with food works well. Liquid vitamin C is usually available at health stores, and many pets take it readily. Use Pau d'Arco extract (3–5 drops PO every 12 hours) either as the alcohol extract or with alcohol removed.[60] Pycnogenol (15 mg PO every 24 hours) and echinacea (3–5 drops PO every 12 hours) may also be of benefit to strengthen the immune system.[18,60]

For clinically ill lymphoma patients in which chemotherapy is not an option because of the patient's condition or client's compliance, administer prednisone (0.5 mg/kg PO every 12 hours) and increase the dose as needed to control clinical signs.[60] Prednisone therapy may be useful in alleviating some of the signs temporarily, improving the quality of life.

It is important to obtain a routine WBC count, even of young animals (older than 6 months), in order to detect lymphoma early enough that hemotherapy can be useful. This disease is frequently overlooked. Because of the probability that this disease is viral in origin, monitor all ferrets in any multiferret household containing a ferret with lymphoma with at least annual CBC counts.

Rabies virus

Since 1958, only 23 ferrets have been reported to the Centers for Disease Control and Prevention as positive for the rabies virus in the United States.[145] Rabies should be considered in any patient with neurologic signs and a history of possible contact with wildlife. Common clinical signs of rabies include ascending paralysis, ataxia, bladder atony, cachexia, fever, hyperactivity, and tremors.[146] Rabies is almost always fatal, although there have been rare cases of recovery.[145] In most other carnivore species studied, rabies is usually transmitted by contact between saliva from an infected, clinically ill animal and the bloodstream of another. In a study of ferrets experimentally infected with the raccoon strain of rabies virus, only one animal from the group of 50 had virus particles present in the submaxillary salivary gland, and none was found in the saliva.[145] However, in any situation involving a rabies suspect, it is recommended that the affected animal be euthanized and the brain submitted for confirmation.[130]

Prevention is provided by proper vaccination and limiting exposure to wildlife. (See chapter 3, Preventative Health Program.)

Splenomegaly

Splenomegaly is a common nonspecific finding in ferrets 2 years of age and older. It is rare to find a ferret older than 2 years that has a "normal"-sized spleen (one that is the size found in a 1-year-old ferret, approximately 5.1 cm in length, 1.8 cm in width, and 0.8 cm in thickness).[7] The spleen is easily palpated in the left cranial abdominal region, parallel to the greater curvature of the stomach.[7] It is readily visualized on a radiograph on the left side of the abdomen as a rectangular organ stretching from the area of the stomach on the left to the middle to lower abdomen. Primary disease of the spleen is uncommon. Histologically, the most common finding in enlarged spleens is extramedullary hematopoiesis. A spleen that increases rapidly in size over a short period of time or is irregular in shape, painful, or so large that it interferes with normal abdominal function (takes up over 50% of the abdominal space) is of immediate concern.

A differential list for primary splenic disease includes the following: lymphoma, hemangiosarcoma, hemangioma, metastatic disease, hematopoietic disease (Aleutian), splenitis, and idiopathic hypersplenism. Idiopathic hypersplenism is a poorly defined disease syndrome seen rarely in ferrets.

The cause of splenomegaly is determined on the basis of a variety of diagnostic tests including a CBC count, Aleutian test, splenic aspirate (see chapter 4, Clinical Techniques), serum biochemistries, and exploratory surgery with splenic biopsy.

Tuberculosis

Classic pulmonary tuberculosis (TB) is a rare disease in the ferret, most commonly seen in the feral population in New Zealand.[147] Ferrets are susceptible to both *Mycobacterium bovis* and *M. avium*.[116] The source is usually ingestion of contaminated raw meat, poultry, or dairy products.

Clinical signs of TB are primarily related to granulomatous enteritis and include anorexia, vomiting, weight loss, debilitation, and diarrhea.[148] The disease invades the mesenteric and abdominal lymph nodes and may lead to emaciation and paralysis of the adductor muscles of the pelvic limbs.[147] The differential diagnosis should include proliferative enteritis, salmonellosis, parasites, GI foreign bodies, and neoplasia. The diagnosis is based on palpation of the enlarged mesenteric lymph nodes and the demonstration of acid-fast bacilli in a lymph node biopsy. No treatment is available at this time, and euthanasia is recommended because of the zoonotic potential for

young, old, and immunosuppressed members of the human
population.

Musculoskeletal System

Hind limb weakness is a common presenting sign in ill ferrets. It is
often nonspecific, and weakness must be differentiated from true neurologic disease. The most common cause of hind limb weakness is
systemic disease and can include a host of problems related to hypoglycemia, anemia, high fevers, malnutrition, oxygen deprivation, and
metabolic imbalance. Some diseases to consider are cardiomyopathy,
insulinoma, adrenal neoplasia, diabetes mellitus, aplastic anemia,
influenza, eosinophilic gastroenteritis, hepatic and renal disease, pneumonia, and wasting diseases such as lymphoma, Aleutian disease, and
GI foreign bodies. Neurologic causes of hind limb weakness include
intervertebral disk disease, hemivertebrae, spinal or pelvic trauma or
fractures, and CNS diseases.

The majority of musculoskeletal problems seen in private practice
involve trauma (e.g., fractures and dislocations). Spinal fractures
should be treated immediately as in other domestic species, with
parenteral corticosteroids, cage rest, and supportive care. Surgical
repair should be considered where appropriate. Limb fractures and
dislocations are treated as in the dog and cat. (See chapter 6,
Orthopedic—Procedure.)

Hemivertebrae occur occasionally as a congenital defect in the ferret.
The malformed vertebra represents a weakened area in the spine, and
the possibility exists for pinching or severing of the spinal cord if the
pet is exposed to any trauma. The diagnosis is based on radiography.

Several types of neoplasia have been found in the ferret skeletal system. Chondrosarcomas, chondromas, chordomas, and osteomas have
been reported.[29,72] Chondromas are benign neoplasms of chondrocytes
usually seen on flat bones.[29] Fibrosarcomas can also arise in bone.[60] A
synovial sarcoma of the stifle has also been seen.[149] Diagnosis and

treatment vary with presentation. Chordomas are aggressive neoplasms arising from primitive notochord elements with moderate metastatic potential.[29] Chordomas are commonly seen on the tip of the tail in older ferrets but can develop anywhere along the spinal vertebrae[29,150] (figure 32). The tail chordoma may become very large and multilobular, and the tumor may become abraded and ulcerated. Chordomas are surgically removed by amputating the portion of the tail containing the tumor. Neoplastic growth in the cervical spine has been reported.[151] Chordomas arising anywhere else on the spine have a poor prognosis because of their metastatic potential.[29]

Neurologic Disorders

Congenital abnormalities of the central nervous system have been reported in the ferret. Neural tube defects were seen in one litter and reported in another with the same sire.[152] Other abnormalities have been discussed anecdotally, but no reports are available.

Intervertebral disk disease (IVD) occurs in the ferret. Onset of signs is often related to a history of trauma. The primary sign is an acute hind limb paresis or paralysis. IVD is diagnosed on the basis of clinical signs and radiographic evidence of narrowing of the disk space or misalignment of the vertebrae. In some cases, because of the small size of the patient, narrowing of the disk space may be difficult to ascertain. A myelogram should be obtained to outline the lesion more clearly. (See chapter 4, Clinical Techniques.) The disease is treated as for the canine patient, using corticosteroid therapy. Physical therapy after acute treatment should include daily swimming in warm water. Clients should be trained in long-term care, including expressing the bladder and proper care of the skin to avoid urine scald and chafing. Many clients have devised support apparatus utilizing carpet glides or wheels for increased ambulation.

Lymphoma can invade the spinal canal and cause pressure on the spinal cord with resulting neurologic signs. This is difficult to diag-

ose and may require a combination of plain radiography, myelogra-
hy, and spinal fluid analysis showing high numbers of lymphocytes.
A granular cell tumor in the brain has also been reported.[153]

eizures in ferrets older than 2 years are primarily caused by
nsulinoma-induced hypoglycemia. The differential diagnosis for
eizures in ferrets includes rabies, canine distemper, head trauma,
eoplasia, septicemia, encephalitis, listeriosis, toxoplasmosis, hepatic
lisease (hepatic encephalopathy), hypoadrenocorticism, GI foreign
ody (due to electrolyte imbalance), high fevers, CNS parasites
(*Baylisascaris procyonis*), and toxin ingestion.[18,44,154] The treatment is
ased on the diagnosis.

'errets have also presented with head tilts.[18] The differential diagnosis
or a head tilt in a ferret includes trauma, otitis interna, CNS parasites,
eoplasia, and inflammatory disease. The treatment is based on the
liagnosis.

phthalmic Disorders

Jnlike other domestic animals, ferrets have immature visual systems
t birth. The eyes do not open until 28 days of age.[8]

Microophthalmia has been reported.[154] The retina has a large number
f cones and ganglion cells, although evidence to date indicates only
n ability to detect the color red.[8] More research into the ferret's abil-
ty to see color is needed. Ferrets use little binocular vision, depending
n monocular vision.[155] Ferrets also have an accessory visual pathway
inked to the pineal gland, believed to be necessary in the link between
he onset of estrus and photoperiod.[8]

Anatomically, the ferret eye is similar to the canine eye, except for the
orizontally slit pupil.[155] Ophthalmoscopic examination reveals a fun-
lus similar to that of the canine.[155] A fundic examination is performed
n an awake ferret in a darkened room with the ophthalmoscope set on
lack 8 for the best results. Dilation of the pupil is seldom necessary.

Blindness

Ferrets can exhibit vision loss caused by cataracts, trauma, congenital abnormality, inflammation, infection, and so forth. Because ferrets naturally have poor eyesight and do not rely primarily on eyesight for survival, they usually adapt well to visual deficits. Because of the relation to photoperiod, intact female ferrets that become blind no longer have estrous cycles.[155] To adapt the home environment to the blind patient, restrict climbing, do not change the furniture, and supervise interaction with other ferrets to avoid injury. Blind ferrets can occasionally have difficulty eating from a bowl.

Cataracts

Cataracts may be hereditary, usually occurring in the first year, or a side effect of aging, possibly influenced by genetic, nutritional, and/or environmental factors.[156] Trauma, diabetes mellitus, and vitamin A or E deficiency have also been implicated in cataract formation.[154,155,157] Cataracts usually occur in both eyes and progress rapidly to blindness. The only known treatment for cataracts is surgical removal. Referral to a veterinary ophthalmologist is recommended.

Cataracts can induce uveitis, as seen in the dog.[157] Clinical signs include miosis, corneal edema, and squinting.[155] Untreated uveitis can lead to glaucoma. Treatment involves topical corticosteroids (1% prednisolone acetate every 12–24 hours, increased to every 6–8 hours if severe) in acute disease.[155] For chronic uveitis, a nonsteroidal anti-inflammatory medication (flurbiprofen or suprofen) is recommended.[155] Ideally, surgical removal of the cataracts will cure the problem.

One possible sequela of cataracts is lens luxation. Although this has been associated more often with retinal atrophy, it can happen in a cataract-affected lens.[156] The signs of anterior lens displacement can be acute, with pain, swelling, and pawing of the eye, as well as pain-induced anorexia. An anteriorly luxated lens requires emergency surgery, either lens removal or removal of the entire eye.[157] Do not dilate the eye before surgery.[157] Sometimes the lens is only partially displaced or displaced into the vitreal chamber, and treatment depends on discomfort to the patient. As an alternative treatment for lens displacement, the globe can be injected under anesthesia with 0.1 cc of full-strength gentamicin.[18] If necessary, the procedure is repeated in 2 weeks.[18] The resultant scarring and shrinking of the eye obviate the need for surgery. Analgesics may be used for several days after treatment for temporary discomfort.[18]

Conjunctivitis

Conjunctivitis in ferrets is most commonly seen with canine distemper virus or influenza. Clinical signs include chemosis, crusting, and mucopurulent discharge, progressing to corneal ulceration or keratoconjunctivitis sicca.[155] The differential diagnosis includes glaucoma, trauma-induced corneal ulcer, ocular foreign bodies, meibomian gland abscesses, distichiasis, and vitamin A deficiency.[155] Schirmer's tear test, fluorescein staining, tonometry, and bacterial culture are used to reach a diagnosis. Bacterial conjunctivitis and corneal ulcers are treated with topical ophthalmic antibiotics as in the dog and cat.

Bacterial conjunctivitis (ophthalmia neonatorum) is seen in kits 12 to 21 days of age.[20] Clinical signs include swelling of the eyelid caused by the accumulation of pus in the conjunctival sac and anorexia. Treat by cutting along the suture line of the eyelids with a scalpel or 25-gauge needle to provide drainage.[20] Apply a broad-spectrum ophthalmic antibiotic ointment once or twice to cure the infection.[20]

Epiphora

Epiphora can be a sign of dental disease of the canines and upper premolars, ocular foreign body, eyelid or eyelash disorders, corneal ulceration, lacrimal duct obstruction, or pain elsewhere in the face or skull. In cases of epiphora without obvious cause, a high-detail skull radiograph is recommended. Fluorescein dye can help rule out corneal disease and lacrimal duct obstructions.

Retinal atrophy

Retinal atrophy involves degeneration and loss of retinal structure, ultimately leading to blindness.[158] In ferrets, the etiology is unknown, but it has been hypothesized to be congenital or diet related.[159] Clinical signs include varying degrees of blindness, usually bilateral, with a hyperreflective retina and avascular fundus on ophthalmoscopic examination.[158,159] There is no treatment for this condition.[158] Intact animals with retinal atrophy should be neutered in the event that it is congenital in origin.

Respiratory System

Introduction

Ferrets normally sneeze and cough loudly and forcefully, which can be alarming to the novice owner. They depend on their sense of smell more than on their eyesight and are constantly inhaling small particles of foreign debris. Occasional sneezing or coughing on a daily basis is entirely normal behavior. If the sneezing is frequent but not associated with any other behavioral changes, an environmental irritant should be investigated. Items such as carpet-deodorizing powders, floor-cleaning solutions, perfumed detergents, or fabric softeners used on cage, bedding, or toys; perfumed clay kitty litter; or cedar shavings can cause chronic sneezing. Placement of the cage near an outflow vent for the furnace or air conditioner can be another source of respiratory irritants. Antihistamines such as chlorpheniramine or diphenhydramine may be useful to control excessive sneezing temporarily, but treatment should be aimed at eliminating the source of the problem.

Influenza

The most common infectious cause of respiratory disease in the ferret is the human influenza virus (Orthomyxoviridae).[130] Transmission is via inhalation of aerosolized viral particles from an infected ferret or human.[134,160] It should be noted that ferrets can also transmit this disease directly to humans. The disease is usually mild and self-limiting

n otherwise healthy adult animals, but it can be fatal in neonates.
Clinical signs of influenza include serous ocular discharge, rhinitis,
anorexia, listlessness, sneezing, coughing, and occasionally diarrhea
and may last from 7 to 14 days.[130,161] The patient may exhibit a
fluctuating temperature of 104 to 105°F (40 to 40.5°C).[130,161] The
differential diagnosis includes canine distemper virus, pulmonary
mycoses, and neoplasia.

A transient leukopenia may be noted in a CBC count. A presumptive
diagnosis is based on clinical signs and history of exposure to infected
individuals.[134] A definite diagnosis can be made by isolation of the
virus from nasal secretions and a rising antibody titer.[134] Supportive
treatment is administered, with restricted exercise, oral fluids, and
assisted feedings. The signs of influenza are controlled with antihistamines such as chlorpheniramine (1–2 mg/kg PO every 8–12 hours) or
diphenhydramine (0.5–2 mg/kg PO every 8–12 hours).[161] The antiviral
medication amantadine (6 mg/kg PO every 12 hours) has been effective in ferret influenza treatment.[134] Antibiotics should be used only if
secondary bacterial infection is suspected. Patients that exhibit recurrent bouts of upper respiratory infection should be screened for
lymphoma with a CBC count (see Lymphoma for more information).
Anyone handling ferrets who exhibits signs of influenza should use a
mask and wash the hands frequently or use disposable gloves to avoid
infecting patients in the hospital.

Pneumonia

Pneumonia is seen occasionally in ferrets. Bacterial agents reported in
ferret pneumonia include *Streptococcus zooepidemicus*, *S.*
pneumoniae, *Escherichia coli*, *Klebsiella pneumoniae*, *Pseudomonas*
aeruginosa, *Listeria monocytogenes,* and *Bordetella bronchiseptica*.[116]
These are usually secondary to canine distemper virus or influenza.[134]
Aspiration pneumonia related to assisted or tube feeding or secondary
to megaesophagus also occurs. Clinical signs include general depression, nasal discharge, anorexia, fever, coughing, and mild to severe

dyspnea.[116] The differential diagnosis includes pulmonary mycoses, heartworm disease, cardiovascular disease, neoplasia, and malignant hyperthermia.[116] Ferrets with pneumonia often exhibit elevated WBC counts of 20,000 x 10^3/µl or higher, with a significant left shift. Radiographs reveal alveolar patterns consistent with pneumonia in other animals.[134] A tracheal wash should be performed with culture and cytology (see chapter 4, Clinical Techniques). Treat with broad-spectrum antibiotics such as cephalosporins, chloramphenicol, or trimethoprim-sulfa. Nebulization with mucolytic agents or antibiotics may aid respiration.

Pulmonary mycoses

Pulmonary mycoses are rare in pet ferrets; however, aspergillosis, cryptococcosis, blastomycosis, histoplasmosis, coccidioidomycosis, and actinomycosis have been reported.[134,162] *Pneumocystis carinii* is now classified as a fungal organism and can cause pulmonary disease in immunocompromised ferrets.[130] Ferrets housed outdoors are at greater risk for contracting mycotic disease.[162] Clinical signs of pulmonary mycoses include sneezing, coughing, weight loss, lethargy, anorexia, and ocular and nasal discharge.[134,162] The differential diagnosis includes bacterial pneumonia, canine distemper virus, influenza, neoplasia, metabolic disease, thoracic trauma, cardiac disease, pulmonary abscesses, and diaphragmatic hernia.[134] Leukocytosis may be noted.[162] Radiographs usually reveal a diffuse pattern consistent with interstitial pneumonia.[162] Perform cytology and bacterial and fungal cultures using a tracheal or lung wash for the definitive diagnosis.[134,162] Treatment is with long-term antifungal therapy as described for the dog and cat.[162] The prognosis for pulmonary mycoses is poor.[134]

Respiratory tract neoplasia

Lymphosarcoma, thymoma, and metastasis of other types of neoplasia occur in the ferret. Respiratory signs range from none to coughing and

yspnea. Diagnosis of these diseases is based on a combination of
adiography and thoracic fluid or thoracic mass cytology or biopsy.

rogenital System

ystitis

rimary cystitis is an uncommon condition in ferrets. It occurs most
requently as an infection secondary to cystic calculus formation, neo-
lasia, or paraurethral cysts in males. Signs include frequent and often
ainful urination. There may be urine staining in the perineal and
nguinal areas (this urine staining may occur normally in intact ani-
nals that are sexually active). The presence of a thick, green,
enacious discharge of the prepuce indicates the presence of
araurethral cysts. The bladder wall is thickened on palpation. Diagnois of cystitis is based on clinical signs and urinalysis. Radiography
nd ultrasonography are useful for ruling out cystic calculi and para-
rethral cysts. Treatment is based on urine culture and sensitivity.
ntibiotic therapy should be used for a minimum of 2 weeks and the
iet corrected as described in the discussion of urolithiasis.

ystocia

formal gestation in the ferret is approximately 42 days. Dystocia is
sually due to uterine inertia, protracted labor (greater than 3 hours),
n overlarge fetus, or a retained placenta. Any or all of these condi-
ions are an indication for an emergency cesarean section (see
hapter 6). If a kit is partially through the birth canal, gentle traction
fter using a water-soluble lubricant may aid delivery.

strogen-induced aplastic anemia (hyperestrogenism)

his condition occurs in the intact female ferret in prolonged
strus.[19,163] Because ferrets are induced ovulators, estrus continues
ntil the ferret is bred, when ovulation is stimulated by pressure on the
ervix.[5] Photoperiod changes (the shortening of the day cycle) also
nd estrus.[5] Ferrets can stay in estrus for 6 months or longer, maintain-

ing consistently high estrogen levels.[5] The high estrogen level can lead to toxic bone marrow suppression, resulting in a nonregenerative anemia that is eventually fatal.[19] Any ferret in estrus for 2 weeks or longer is at risk. Clinical signs of aplastic anemia include anorexia, vulvar swelling, vulvar discharge, depression, hind limb weakness, lethargy, and pale mucous membranes.[164] Petechiae and ecchymoses may be present on the mucous membranes and skin.[164] Females in prolonged estrus may also develop a bilaterally symmetrical alopecia1[164] (figure 27). Clinical signs are not usually evident until the PCV is less than 20% and/or the platelet count is less than 50,000/mm^3.[163] Hematology reveals a severe nonregenerative anemia, normocytic RBCs, nucleated RBCs, depressed PCV (less than 25%), neutropenia, and thrombocytopenia.[5,165]

To take a ferret out of estrus safely, several options have been suggested, including a vasectomized male, mechanical stimulation, and chemical alteration of the hormonal system. A vasectomized male ferret can be used to bring females out of estrus and into pseudopregnancy, but the results are variable and unpredictable.[166] The use of cotton-tipped applicators or other products to stimulate the female mechanically has been unsuccessful. Chemical methods include human chorionic gonadotropin (hCG) (100 IU per ferret IM) at least 10 days after the onset of estrus.[166] If there has been no response in 2 weeks, repeat the dose. Alternatively, gonadotropin-releasing hormone (GnRH) (20 µg per ferret SC or IM) may be used.[164] Repeated use of hCG or GnRH may stimulate antibody formation and resistance. Neither hCG nor GnRH will terminate estrus if the ferret has been in heat for a prolonged time (a month or longer), and ovariohysterectomy (OVH) may be necessary. Do not use progesterone products with intact ferrets because pyometra may result.

Because severe leukopenia, thrombocytopenia, and anemia may result from prolonged estrous periods, a CBC and platelet count should be obtained for any patient in estrus for 2 weeks or longer prior to any

rgery or other therapy. If the ferret shows signs of bone marrow sup-
ression, an OVH is advised. The PCV, combined with the RBC and
latelet counts and differential, is used to indicate the severity of dis-
ase. If the PCV is greater than 25%, the prognosis is guarded to good
nd termination of estrus is often successful. PCVs between 15 and
5% result in a guarded to poor prognosis. If the PCV is less than
5%, the prognosis is poor and treatment with multiple blood transfu-
ons is often unsuccessful.[165] Euthanasia is necessary if the patient
oes not respond to therapy or the RBC parameters are inconsistent
ith recovery. Ferrets can receive multiple blood transfusions, from
ultiple donors, as they have no apparent blood type[36] (see chapter 4).

complex vitamins, anabolic steroids, antibiotics, fluid therapy, and
ssisted feedings are all appropriate therapy at this stage. The progno-
s for severe estrogen-induced aplastic anemia is guarded to grave
ecause of the persistently high estrogen levels for up to 6 weeks after
VH. An OVH at this point may be fatal, despite the necessity. The
est course of action is prevention by spaying female ferrets at 4 to
months of age or within 2 weeks of the first estrus. A CBC and
latelet count should always be obtained before performing an OVH
n any ferret who has been in estrus for 2 weeks or longer to deter-
ine whether bone marrow suppression has already occurred. If the
BC and/or platelet count indicate abnormalities, supportive care such
anabolic steroids, erythropoietin, and transfusions should be given
ostsurgically.

eutered female ferrets who show signs of coming back into
strus (enlarged vulva or hair loss) are affected with either adrenal-
ssociated endocrinopathy (see Endocrine System) or remnant ovarian
ssue. The remnant tissue may be normal and present at the ovarian
ump or ectopically located in the mesenteric fat. Cystic ovarian rem-
ants have been reported in spayed ferrets.[167] Neoplasia of ovarian
mnants, such as luteoma and granulosa cell tumor, has also been
ported.[18] Treatment involves removal of the abnormal tissue found
abdominal exploratory surgery (see chapter 6).

Hydronephrosis

Hydronephrosis has been reported in the ferret.[18,168] All cases reported thus far have been iatrogenic, secondary to OVH. Clinical signs of advanced disease can include polyuria and polydipsia, vomiting, lethargy, anorexia, and melena. The affected kidney is enlarged on palpation. The differential diagnosis includes polycystic kidney disease and neoplasia. A CBC count, blood chemistries, and a urinalysis are used to determine renal function. Abdominal ultrasonography or intravenous pyelography (IVP) reveals the diagnosis. Surgical removal of the affected kidney is the treatment of choice.

Mastitis

Mastitis is caused by damage to the mammary gland with secondary invasion by opportunistic bacteria.[169] Most cases occur when kits are about 3 weeks old (when the teeth erupt), with exceptionally large litters, or when a rough edge on the opening to the nest damages the mammary glands.[169] Clinical signs of mastitis include multilobular, firm, painful, often discolored mammary glands; depression; fever; pulmonary rales; nasal discharge; diarrhea; and anorexia.[19,20] The diagnosis is based on clinical signs. Treat with appropriate antibiotics on the basis of culture and sensitivity results for milk expressed from affected glands. Treatment is usually with a broad-spectrum antibiotic.[20] The addition of flunixin meglumine or carprofen reduces pain, improves recovery, and decreases inflammation.[18,20] The character of mastitis depends on the infective organism. *Staphylococcus* spp. infections can become chronic, decreasing milk availability and nutrition to the kits.[20] *Escherichia coli* can cause acute gangrenous mastitis in ferrets.[20] Mortality is common with *E. coli* infection because of the release of endotoxins into the bloodstream.[19] In some cases, wide surgical excision of the affected gland(s) is necessary for the survival of the jill. Supportive care includes subcutaneous fluids, high-protein, high-fat liquid diets, and supplementation of the kits with warmed milk replacer at least three times daily.[20] Mastitis in ferrets can be ontagious to other nursing jills, and careful sanitation and segregation of affected ferrets are necessary.[20,169] Ferrets severely affected by mastitis should be spayed because of a permanently decreased milk supply and to prevent recurrence.

Metritis

Retention of a kit or placental attachment can lead to metritis.[169] This condition can be fatal if left untreated. Signs of metritis include depression, fever, and anorexia, with or without a dark red vaginal discharge.[20,169] The uterus is enlarged on abdominal palpation. Diagnosis is based on history and clinical signs. A culture and sensitivity test of the uterus should be performed if the cervix is open. Treatment is with an appropriate antibiotic and prostaglandin F_{2a}. Aggressive supportive care should include fluid therapy, highly palatable high-protein, high-fat supplements for the jill, and milk replacer for the kits.[20,169] Trimethoprim-sulfa combinations are recommended to prevent ascending urinary tract disease.[20] NSAIDs such as flunixin and carprofen aid in recovery, but prostaglandin antagonists should be avoided during prostaglandin F_{2a} use.[20] OVH is the treatment of choice. The prognosis for future fertility is guarded.

Paraurethral cysts

Male ferrets older than 3 years can develop an enlargement of the prostatic tissue surrounding the urethra. The enlargement can be due to infection, cyst formation, and/or inflammation.[42] Paraurethral cysts have been seen most often secondary to adrenal-associated endocrinopathy and may be caused by the effects of excess androgens produced by the adrenal glands[164,168] (see Endocrine System). Clinical signs of paraurethral cysts are consistent with urinary tract obstruction and include dysuria, tenacious green preputial discharge, and crying upon urination. A mass is palpable dorsal to the bladder on physical examination. The differential diagnosis includes cystic calculi and neoplasia. A CBC count and serum biochemistries determine concurrent renal disease, acidosis, and other metabolic abnormalities.

Urinalysis may reveal a leukocytosis. Radiography reveals a soft-tissue density within or anterior to the pelvis and dorsal to the bladder and rules out urolithiasis (figure 17). Ultrasound examination definitively identifies the paraurethral enlargement, as well as other abdominal abnormalities. A presumptive diagnosis of adrenal-associated endocrinopathy with secondary paraurethral cyst formation is based on history, clinical signs, and physical examination.

The treatment of choice is surgical removal of the affected adrenal gland(s) (see chapter 6). Urinary catheterization or cystocentesis (see chapter 4) may be necessary to relieve the bladder before surgery. If the cyst(s) is large, reduction by surgical debulking may be helpful, but removal of the prostatic tissue is usually not necessary. Obtain a bacterial culture and sensitivity test of the contents after drainage. If necessary, marsupialization of the cyst to the abdominal or bladder wall will allow drainage. Fluid therapy and analgesics should be administered as needed. Treat with antibiotics if infection is found. Normal urination usually occurs 3 to 5 days after surgery.

If surgery is not an option, pressure on the bladder can be relieved by catheterization or cystocentesis (see chapter 4). Surgical placement of a cystotomy tube is an option if catheterization is unsuccessful (see chapter 6). Administer fluid therapy and electrolytes as needed on the basis of blood abnormalities. Treat with antibiotics on the basis of culture and sensitivity of the preputial discharge or aspirated contents of paraurethral cysts. Corticosteroids or other anti-inflammatory analgesics may be necessary for immediate relief of pain and inflammation. Flutamide (10 mg/kg PO every 12–24 hours) has proved efficacious in decreasing prostatic tissue enlargement in the long term. Treatment with flutamide is less successful in cases with complete urinary obstruction. Use of flutamide is lifelong (see Endocrine System).

There is a high rate of recurrence of paraurethral cyst(s), especially in cases with unilateral adrenalectomy or nonsurgical candidates. It is

ecessary to monitor these patients closely with physical examinations
t 3- to 4-month intervals.

regnancy toxemia

'regnancy toxemia usually occurs when a late-term jill is fasted or
vhen she is carrying a very large litter.[20] Clinical signs include
nelena, lethargy, dehydration, anorexia, and heavy shedding.[20] Abnor-
nalities in the diagnostic blood tests include a PCV less than 30%,
ypoglycemia, and azotemia. Ketonuria can be found on
rinalysis.[19,20] An immediate cesarean section should be performed if
he jill is between days 39 and 41 of pregnancy. Aggressive supportive
are should be used, including IV fluids, antibiotics, and high-protein
nd high-fat diet supplements. Performing surgery any earlier in the
regnancy will result in loss of the kits but may be necessary to save
he life of the jill. See chapter 2 for dietary methods for preventing
regnancy toxemia.

rimary renal disease

'rimary renal disease is not commonly reported in the ferret, but it
nay be underdiagnosed because of the tendency of the North Ameri-
an ferret to develop other diseases and continuing controversy over
ormal serum biochemistry renal values. Clinical signs may include
norexia, foul odor of the breath, oral ulcerations, depression, polyuria
nd polydipsia, melena, hind limb weakness, fever, and severe dehy-
ration.[19,164] Small, irregular kidneys, pale mucous membranes, and
achexia may be found on physical examination. The differential diag-
osis includes pyelonephritis, progressive renal failure, chronic
nterstitial nephritis (usually found at postmortem examination),
lomerulonephropathy secondary to Aleutian disease, neoplasia,
ydronephrosis, and polycystic kidney disease.[19,164] Urinalysis reveals
sosthenuria, casts, bactiuria, and/or leukocytes in the urine.[19] A CBC
ount shows nonregenerative anemia in long-term kidney disease.[164]
erum biochemistry values in ferrets differ from those in dogs and
ats with renal insufficiency. The creatinine level frequently does not

rise above normal, even in ferrets with clinical signs of renal disease.[105,141] However, there is still controversy over the normal creatinine range in the ferret, and this issue has not been resolved at the time of this writing. Elevated creatinine is an indicator of severe and long-term kidney malfunction.[105] Elevations in blood urea nitrogen (BUN) and phosphorus are diagnostic indicators of renal insufficiency.[105] Radiographs indicate size changes in the kidneys. Ultrasonography with or without renal biopsy can give a definitive diagnosis.

Treatment is similar to that used for canine and feline patients. Administer IV or IO fluid therapy for correction of electrolyte and fluid balance abnormalities, antibiotics for infection, erythropoietin for anemia, and phosphorus-binding agents to reduce serum phosphorus levels. Although protein may be reduced slightly, it should still be maintained in the diet at 32%. The quality of the protein is more important in reducing the renal workload. The patient should be maintained with a high-quality, meat-based protein and high-fat source to maintain muscle mass, weight, and energy. The prognosis is guarded to poor.

Pyometra

Pyometra can occur in the intact female as a result of ascending infections of the vagina, retained fetuses, and blood-borne infectious agents. Iatrogenic pyometra can be caused by prostaglandin or progesterone products administered to an intact female. Clinical signs of pyometra include depression, anorexia, fever, and lethargy, with or without a vaginal discharge.[19,64] The differential diagnosis includes estrogen-induced aplastic anemia (which may be present concurrently) and metritis. A CBC count may show a neutrophilic leukocytosis.[64] Enlarged uterine horns may be visible on abdominal radiographs. The treatment of choice is OVH (see chapter 6). The uterine wall should be cultured for appropriate postsurgical antibiotic therapy.

tump pyometra has been reported in a spayed ferret.[170] Pyometra has
lso been seen in ovarian remnants with uterine tissue attached.[18] The
resenting complaint was alopecia of the dorsal lumbar area and tail,
vith polyuria, polydipsia, and poor litterbox habits.[170] Clinical signs
ncluded vomiting, lethargy, and anorexia with fever.[170] Physical
xamination revealed a slightly enlarged vulva and a palpable enlarged
nass in the caudal abdomen, from which mucopurulent material was
spirated.[170] Radiography may show a caudal abdominal mass. Surgi-
al removal with supportive care is curative. Antibiotic therapy should
e instituted on the basis of culture and sensitivity. Cystic enlargement
f the uterine stump, with or without infection, has been associated
vith adrenal disease.[18,164]

enal cysts

ystic kidney disease can occur in the ferret at any age.[18] Polycystic
isease is hypothesized to be due to a benign congenital abnormality,
nd cystic disease is secondary to an ascending urinary tract
nfection.[171] Clinical signs are noted only in the event of renal insuffi-
iency and include lethargy, inappetence, vomiting, pu/pd, and
nelena.[168] Enlarged, irregular kidneys are noted during physical
xamination. In cystic kidney disease, the enlargement is smooth,
ends to be more pronounced at the anterior pole, and can be unilateral
r bilateral. Polycystic kidneys are found in ferrets younger than
 year of age and are enlarged and very irregular (lumpy). The differ-
ntial diagnosis includes neoplasia and hydronephrosis. A CBC count,
erum biochemistries, and urinalysis aid in determining renal function.
bdominal ultrasonography can differentiate cystic kidneys from other
isorders. No treatment is necessary if renal function is unimpaired.
he progression should be monitored via blood chemistries, urinalysis,
nd ultrasonography at regular intervals. If the condition is unilateral
nd the affected kidney becomes greatly enlarged, nephrectomy is the
reatment of choice.[168]

Reproductive tract neoplasms

Reproductive tract neoplasms are seldom seen in private practice in the United States because of the practice of early neutering. Reported neoplasms in the reproductive tract of the ferret include granulosa cell tumor, luteoma, uterine leiomyoma, ovarian thecoma, uterine and ovarian teratomas, uterine adenoma, undifferentiated carcinoma of the ovarian stump, cystic carcinoma of the mammary gland, and fibrosarcoma in the female.[59,60,72] Male ferrets are prone to Sertoli cell and interstitial cell tumors; a seminoma and carcinoma of the prostate have also been reported.[60,72] Clinical signs of reproductive tract neoplasm vary, depending on the site and level of hormone production involved. Neoplasia of the reproductive tract of the male and the female may lead to generalized alopecia. Clinical signs, physical examination, and radiographs lead to the diagnosis. Surgical removal is the treatment of choice. Chemotherapy or radiation therapy is indicated where appropriate.

Urinary tract neoplasms

Renal adenocarcinomas cause the surface of the kidney to feel irregular and very "lumpy" on palpation. Lymphoma, papillary tubular cystadenoma, and transitional cell carcinoma have also been reported in the ferret kidney.[60,103] Radiographs demonstrate these irregularities, and often the affected kidney appears denser than the unaffected one. Ultrasonography with or without biopsy may be necessary for a definitive diagnosis.[60] A nephrectomy is advised if neoplasia is suspected.[60] The surgical procedure for kidney removal in the ferret is the same as in the cat.

Transitional cell carcinoma has been reported in the bladder of the ferret.[60] Clinical signs include hematuria, dysuria or polyuria, and incontinence.[60] Abnormalities of the bladder may be palpable on physical examination. Urinalysis reveals abnormally large numbers of transitional cells, some abnormal.[60] Radiography is seldom diagnostic without contrast procedures.[60] Ultrasonography may detect a lesion in the bladder. Definitive diagnosis is often via biopsy during abdominal exploratory examination. The prognosis is poor.[60]

Urolithiasis

Urolithiasis is seen in the ferret and may occur in both male and female patients of any age.[19,65] It was very common in pregnant jills in one study.[20] The stones may be solitary or multiple and are usually composed of magnesium ammonium phosphate hexahydrate (struvite).[65,168] Stone formation may be secondary to ascending bacterial infection with agents such as *Staphylococcus* sp. or *Proteus* sp.[19,65] Bell has noted that diets that have high levels of plant protein may predispose ferrets to struvite crystal formation by producing a urine pH over 6.0.[68] There have been reports of cystine calculi of unknown etiology in ferrets.[18,172]

Clinical signs associated with urolithiasis include dysuria, hematuria, frequent urination, crying upon urination, a wet perineum, constant licking of the urogenital opening, and urinary incontinence.[19,68] Occasionally small calculi may be grossly visible in the voided urine. Male (and rarely female) ferrets can present with a complete urinary tract obstruction.[164] Urinary calculi and/or thickening of the bladder wall is palpable on physical examination. The differential diagnosis includes paraurethral cysts in the male, neoplasia, or primary cystitis. A CBC count and serum biochemistries should be performed to determine renal function and electrolyte abnormalities. RBCs, WBCs, and crystals are found on urinalysis. Radiographs reveal calculi in the bladder and possibly the urethra. Ultrasonography can detect the presence of radiolucent stones.

The pressure within the bladder should be relieved immediately. It can be extremely difficult to catheterize a male that has a urinary blockage (see chapter 4). Cystocentesis can temporarily relieve the pressure. Cystocentesis should be performed with the patient under anesthesia to avoid lacerating the bladder. In the obstructed ferret it is usually necessary to perform an emergency cystotomy to remove the calculi and retrograde flush the urethra (see chapter 6). If necessary, place a cystotomy tube or perform a cystopexy (see chapter 6). Perineal urethrostomy can be attempted as a last resort. Cultures should be obtained at the time of surgery and calculi analyzed. Administer concurrent fluid therapy to correct electrolyte imbalances. Treat with broad-spectrum antibiotics if infection is suspected.

Postsurgically, the patient should be given systemic antibiotics for a minimum of 10 to 14 days based on the results of urine culture and sensitivity. In the absence of a urine culture, use a broad-spectrum antibiotic such as amoxicillin or trimethoprim-sulfa.[164] Trials with s/d (Hill's Pet Products, Topeka, KS) have not proven successful in ferrets.[164]

Vaginitis

This disease occurs in jills after the second week of estrus and occasionally in pregnant and postparturient jills.[169] Vaginitis is usually the result of irritation of the vaginal lining, allowing opportunistic bacterial infection.[19] Wood, hay, and straw bedding have been implicated in vaginitis.[19] It is contagious and can be transmitted via vasectomized males used for inducing ovulation.[169] Vaginitis is also seen in neutered females. The etiology of vaginitis in sprites includes dry vaginal tissues or chronically swollen vulva caused by adrenal-associated endocrinopathy; cystitis, crystaluria, or metritis; and exposure to intact males that cause damage to the vagina during mating attempts.[18,19] Clinical signs include a thick yellow to green discharge with little odor, constant licking, necrosis of the outer margins of the vagina and vulva, and occasionally fever.[19,169] Foreign material may be found within the vagina on physical examination.[19] Diagnosis is based on clinical signs and physical examination. *Staphylococcus*, *Proteus* spp., and other enteric bacteria are usually found with culture and sensitivity testing of the vagina.[19,169] Treat with appropriate antibiotics systemically and use hCG or GnRH to interrupt the estrous cycle.[18,169]

Clinical Pathology Values

research is still going on to determine accurate clinical pathology information on the ferret. Do not rely too heavily on these values to diagnose disease, but rather use these data in conjunction with a thorough physical examination, history, and other diagnostic tools as needed to form an overall clinical picture. Work with your own clinical pathology laboratory to develop a list of normal serum or plasma biochemistry values. (See table of ferret biodata in chapter 2.)

Urine

pH: 6.5 to 7.5[9]

Proteinuria: mild to moderate is common and normal[9]

Urine volume: 26 to 28 ml/24-hour average[9]

Feces

Soft, tubular, and formed

Hematologic Values

Blood values, except where noted, based on 40 normal ferrets (6 to 12 months of age, neutered, no clinical evidence of disease and no differentiation by color). Information provided by Antech Diagnostics (Farmingdale, NY 11735).

Blood volume: mature male 60 ml average, mature female 40 ml average (approximately 7–10% body weight)[9,32]

Packed cell volume (PCV): 43–55%

Red blood cells (RBCs) (x 10^6/mm^3): 6.5–11

Hemoglobin (g/dl): 12–18.5

White blood cells (WBCs) (x 10^3/mm^3): 2.5–8

The authors feel that WBC counts greater than 10.0 x 10^3/mm^3
are abnormal.

Neutrophils: 50–80%

Lymphocytes: 20–50%

*Absolute lymphocyte counts over 3500 x 10^3/mm^3 should cause the
practitioner to be suspicious of lymphoma (see chapter 7). Also, in
the authors' opinion, patients with persistent lymphocyte counts
over 60% even in the presence of a low WBC count should be
investigated for lymphoma.

Monocytes: 0–3%

Eosinophils: 0–1%

*An absolute eosinophilia of 800 x 10^3/mm^3 or more may be
indicative of eosinophilic gastroenteritis (see chapter 7).

Basophils: 0–1%

Platelets (10^3/mm^3): 300–750

Serum or Plasma Biochemistry Values

Total protein (g/dl): 5.5–7.6

Albumin (g/dl): 2.4–4.5

Globulin (g/dl): 2.9–4.9

Glucose (fasting):

90–125[18]

up to 207 mg/dl[9] (nonfasting)

Blood urea nitrogen (BUN) (mg/dl): Up to 35[105]

Alkaline phosphatase (IU/L): 15–45

Serum glutamic-oxaloacetic transaminase (SGOT) (IU/L): 50–280

Serum glutamic-pyruvic transaminase (SGPT) (IU/L): 10–280

Total bilirubin (mg/dl): 0–1.0

Creatinine (mg/dl): <0.5[105]

Sodium (mmol/L): 140–160

Potassium (mmol/L): 4.3–5.8

hloride (mmol/L): 90–110

alcium (mg/L): 7.7–11.0

organic phosphorus (mg/dl): 4.0–9.1[9]

O_2: 20–28 MEq/l[9]

holesterol (mg/dl): 60–300

ndocrine Levels: Normal Values

drenal-related hormones from the University of Tennessee Clinical
Endocrinology Laboratory.[82]

ortisol (nmol/L): <140

7-Hydroxyprogesterone (nmol/L): <0.8

stradiol (pmol/L): <180

ndrostenedione (nmol/L): <15

ehydroepiandrosterone sulfate (DHEAS) (nmol/L): <28

sulin (units/ml): 0–20[18]

mol/L): <350[141]

29–387[173]

U/ml): 4–53.9[173]

nsulin values vary greatly between laboratories; it is important to
establish normal values for each laboratory and hospital.

riiodothyronine (T_3) (males): 0.45–0.78 ng/ml[174]
(females): 0.29–0.73 ng/ml

hyroxine (T_4): 1.2–3.8 g/dl (intact males slightly higher)[174]

herapeutic Drug Values

igoxin (ng/ml): 0.8–2.0; extrapolated from dogs and cats[31]

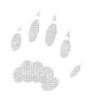

References

. Fox JG. Taxonomy, history and use. In Fox JG, ed. Biology and diseases of the ferret, 2nd ed. Baltimore: Williams & Wilkins, 1998:3–18.

. Macdonald D, ed. The encyclopedia of mammals. New York: Facts on File Publications, 1985:108–29.

. Bell JA. Ferrets—reproduction. In Proceedings of the Small Mammal Conference. Baltimore: American Ferret Association, 1996:1–3.

. Brown SA. Basic anatomy, physiology, and husbandry. In Hillyer EV, Quesenberry KE, eds. Ferrets, rabbits and rodents: clinical medicine and surgery. Philadelphia: WB Saunders, 1997:99–114.

. Fox JG, Bell JA. Growth, reproduction, and breeding. In Fox JG, ed. Biology and diseases of the ferret, 2nd ed. Baltimore: Williams & Wilkins, 1998:211–27.

. Brown SA, Hillyer EV. Dermatologic diseases. In Birchard SJ, Sherding RG, eds. Saunders manual of small animal practice. Philadelphia: WB Saunders, 1994:1332–4.

. Evans HE, An NQ. Anatomy of the ferret. In Fox JG, ed. Biology and diseases of the ferret, 2nd ed. Baltimore: Williams & Wilkins, 1998:19–69.

. Whary MT, Andrews PLR. Physiology of the ferret. In Fox JG, ed. Biology and diseases of the ferret, 2nd ed. Baltimore: Williams & Wilkins, 1998:103–48.

9.   Fox JG. Normal clinical and biologic parameters. In Fox JG, ed. Biology and diseases of the ferret, 2nd ed. Baltimore: Williams & Wilkins, 1998:183–210.

10.   Burgmann PM. Restraint techniques and anaesthetic recommendations for rabbits, rodents, and ferrets. J Small Exotic Anim Med 1991;1(2):73–8.

11.   Morrisey JK, Carpenter JW, Kolmstetter CM. Restraint and diagnostic techniques for ferrets. Vet Med 1996;91:1084–97.

12.   Brown SA. Clinical techniques in domestic ferrets. Seminars in Avian Exotic Pet Med 1997;6(2):75–85.

13.   Hillyer EV, Quesenberry KE. Ferrets: clinical techniques. In Birchard SJ, Sherding RG, eds. Saunders manual of small animal practice. Philadelphia: WB Saunders, 1994:1318–21.

14.   Bell JA. Ensuring proper nutrition in ferrets. Vet Med 1996;91:1098–1103.

15.   Fox JG, McLain DE. Nutrition. In Fox JG, ed. Biology and diseases of the ferret, 2nd ed. Baltimore: Williams & Wilkins, 1998:149–72.

16.   Bell JA. Ferret nutrition & diseases associated with inadequate nutrition. Proc North Am Vet Conf 1993;7:719–20.

17.   Fox JG. Housing and management. In Fox JG, ed. Biology and diseases of the ferret, 2nd ed. Baltimore: Williams & Wilkins, 1998:173–81.

18.   Brown SA. Personal experience.

19.   Fox JG, Pearson RC, Bell JA. Diseases of the genitourinary system. In Fox JG, ed. Biology and diseases of the ferret, 2nd ed. Baltimore: Williams & Wilkins, 1998:247–72.

0. Bell JA. Periparturient and neonatal disease. In Hillyer EV, Quesenberry KE, eds. Ferrets, rabbits and rodents: clinical medicine and surgery. Philadelphia: WB Saunders, 1997:53–62.

1. Peter AT, Bell JA, Manning DD, Bosu WTK. Real-time ultrasonographic determination of pregnancy and gestational age in ferrets. Lab Anim Sci 1990;40:91–2.

2. Smith DA, Burgmann PM. Formulary. In Hillyer EV, Quesenberry KE, eds. Ferrets, rabbits and rodents: clinical medicine and surgery. Philadelphia: WB Saunders, 1997:392–3.

3. Rosenthal KL. Bacterial infections and antibiotic therapy in small mammals. Compendium 1998;20(3A):13–22.

4. Marini RP, Fox JG. Anesthesia, surgery and biomethodology. In Fox JG, ed. Biology and diseases of the ferret, 2nd ed. Baltimore: Williams & Wilkins, 1998:449–84.

5. Quesenberry KE. Basic approach to ferret care. In Hillyer EV, Quesenberry KE, eds. Ferrets, rabbits and rodents: clinical medicine and surgery. Philadelphia: WB Saunders, 1997:14–25.

6. Hoover JP, Baldwin CA, Rupprecht CE. Serologic response of domestic ferrets (*Mustela putorius furo*) to canine distemper and rabies virus vaccines. JAVMA 1989;194:234–8.

7. Rupprecht CE, Gilbert J, Pitts R, Marshall KR, Koprowski H. Evaluation of an inactivated rabies virus vaccine in domestic ferrets. JAVMA 1990;196:1614–16.

8. The National Association of State Public Health Veterinarians (NASPHV). Compendium of animal rabies control, 1998. JAVMA 1998;212:213–17.

9. Williams BH. Personal communication, 1998.

30. Kemmerer D. Ferret heartworm prevention and treatment. Proceedings of the Small Mammal Conference. Baltimore: American Ferret Association, 1996.

31. Stamoulis ME, Miller MS. Cardiovascular diseases. Part I. In Hillyer EV, Quesenberry KE, eds. Ferrets, rabbits and rodents: clinical medicine and surgery. Philadelphia: WB Saunders, 1997:63–70.

32. Fulton LM. Hematology and transfusion medicine in the ferret. Proceedings of the Small Mammal Conference. Baltimore: American Ferret Association, 1996:91.

33. Marini RP, Jackson LR, Esteves MI, Andrutis KA, Goslant CM, Fox JG. Effect of isoflurane on hematologic variables in ferrets. Am J Vet Res 1994;55:1479–83.

34. Ko JCH, Heaton-Jones TG, Nicklin CF. Evaluation of the sedative and cardiorespiratory effects of medetomidine, medetomidine-butorphanol, medetomidine-ketamine, and medetomidine-butorphanol-ketamine in ferrets. JAAHA 1997;33(5):438–48.

35. Erdman S. Venipuncture in the ferret. Proc North Am Vet Conf 1993;7:733.

36. Manning D, Bell J. Lack of detectable blood groups in domestic ferrets: implications for transfusion. JAVMA 1990;197:84–6.

37. Hillyer EV. Blood transfusion techniques in ferrets. Proceedings of the Eastern States Conference, Orlando, 1992:181.

38. Finkler M. Ferrets—blood collection. Proceedings of the Small Mammal Conference. Baltimore: American Ferret Association, 1996:12–13.

9. Bennett RA. Intraosseous catheters in small mammals. Scientific Proceedings, 10th Annual North American Veterinary Conference, Orlando, 1996:847.

10. Palley LS, Marini RP, Rosenbald WD, Fox JG. A technique for femoral bone marrow collection in the ferret. Lab Anim Sci 1990;40:654–5.

11. Marini RP, Esteves MI, Fox JG. A technique for catheterization of the urinary bladder in the ferret. Lab Anim 1994;28:155–7.

12. Bennett RA. Ferret abdominal surgical procedures. Proceedings of the Midwest Exotic Pet Seminars, Oakbrook, IL, 1998.

13. Rubel GA, Isenbugel E, Wolvekamp P. Atlas of diagnostic radiology of exotic pets: small mammals, birds, reptiles and amphibians. Philadelphia: WB Saunders, 1991:9.

14. Hoefer H. Cardiac disease in ferrets. Proceedings of the Midwest Exotic Pet Seminar, Oakbrook, IL, 1998.

15. Antinoff N. Musculoskeletal and neurologic diseases. In Hillyer EV, Quesenberry KE, eds. Ferrets, rabbits and rodents: clinical medicine and surgery. Philadelphia: WB Saunders, 1997:126–30.

16. Rosenthal KL. Adrenal gland disease in ferrets. Vet Clin North Am Small Anim Pract 1997;27:401–18.

17. Miller M. Ferret cardiology. Proc North Am Vet Conf 1993;7:735.

18. Olin JM, Smith TJ, Talcott MR. Evaluation of noninvasive monitoring techniques in domestic ferrets (*Mustela putorius furo*). Am J Vet Res 1997;58:1065–9.

19. Weiss CA, Scott MV. Clinical aspects and surgical treatment of hyperadrenocortism in the domestic ferret: 94 cases (1994–1996). JAAHA 1997;33:487–93.

50. Mason DE. Anesthesia, analgesia, and sedation for small mammals. In Hillyer EV, Quesenberry KE, eds. Ferrets, rabbits and rodents: clinical medicine and surgery. Philadelphia: WB Saunders, 1997:378–91.

51. Heard D. Principles and techniques of anesthesia and analgesia for exotic practice. Vet Clin North Am Small Anim Pract 1993;23:1301–27.

52. Murat I, Housmans P. Minimum alveolar concentrations (MAC) of halothane, enflurane and isoflourane in ferrets. Anesthesiology 1988;68:783–6.

53. Ko JCH, Villarreal A, Kuo W-C, Nicklin CF. Evaluation of sedative and cardiorespiratory effects of diazepam, butorphanol, acepromazine-butorphanol, and xylazine-butorphanol in ferrets. JAAHA 1998;34:242–50.

54. Beeber NJ. Surgery of pet ferrets. In Bojrab MJ, Ellison GW, Slocum B, eds. Current techniques in small animal surgery, 4th ed. Baltimore: Williams & Wilkins, 1998:763–9.

55. Ko JCH, Nicklin CF, Montgomery T, Kuo WC. Comparison of anesthetic and cardiorespiratory effects of tiletamine-zolazepam-xylazine-butorphanol in ferrets. JAAHA 1998;34:164–74.

56. Ko JCH, Nicklin CF, Heaton-Jones TG, Kuo W-C. Comparison of sedative and cardiorespiratory effects of diazepam, acepromazine and xylazine in ferrets. J Am Anim Hosp Assoc 1998;34:234–41.

57. Bennett, RA. Surgical concerns for small exotic animals. Proceedings for the Midwest Exotic Pet Seminar, Oakbrook, IL, 1998.

58. Dutton MA. Hyperadrenocortism in ferrets. Exotic Pet Pract 1997;2(2):9–12.

9. Li X, Fox JG, Padrid PA. Neoplastic disease in ferrets: 574 cases (1968–1997). JAVMA 1998;212:1402–6.

0. Brown SA. Neoplasia. In Hillyer EV, Quesenberry KE, eds. Ferrets, rabbits and rodents: clinical medicine and surgery. Philadelphia: WB Saunders, 1997:99–114.

1. Dutton MA. Personal communication, 1997.

2. Bennett A. Personal communication, 1998.

3. Rosenthal K. Personal communication at the AVMA Convention, Baltimore, 1998.

4. Mullen H. Ferrets: soft tissue surgery. In Hillyer EV, Quesenberry KE, eds. Ferrets, rabbits and rodents: clinical medicine and surgery. Philadelphia: WB Saunders, 1997:131–44.

5. Nguyen HT, Moreland AF, Shields RP. Urolithiasis in ferrets (*Mustela putorius*). Lab Anim Sci 1979;29:243–5.

6. Kyles AE, Stone EA. Cystotomy and cystectomy. In Bojrab MJ, Ellison GW, Slocum B, eds. Current techniques in small animal surgery, 4th ed. Baltimore: Williams & Wilkins, 1998:451–4.

7. Li X, Fox JG, Erdman SE, Lipman NS, Murphy JC. Cystic urogenital anomalies in ferrets (*Mustela putorius furo*). Vet Pathol 1996;33(2):150–8.

8. Bell JA. Management of urinary obstruction in the ferret. Proc North Am Vet Conf 1993;7:724.

9. Rosenthal KL. Ferret endocrine disease: adrenal gland disease and insulinoma disease. Proceedings of the Annual Convention. Baltimore: American Veterinary Medical Association, 1998:594–6.

0. Gates LV. Cystopexy and cystotomy tube placement. Proceedings of the Small Mammal Conference. Baltimore: American Ferret Association, 1997.

71. Weiss CA, Williams BH, Scott MV. Insulinoma in the ferret: clinical findings and treatment. Comparison in 66 cases. JAAHA 1998;34:471–5.

72. Beach JE, Greenwood B. Spontaneous neoplasia in the ferret (*Mustela putorius furo*). J Comp Pathol 1993;108(2):133–47.

73. Kapatkin A. Orthopedics in small mammals. In Hillyer EV, Quesenberry KE, eds. Ferrets, rabbits and rodents: clinical medicine and surgery. Philadelphia: WB Saunders, 1997:346–57.

74. Ryland LM, Lipinski E. A technique for vasectomizing male ferrets. Canine Pract 1994;19(1):25–7.

75. Stamoulis ME. Cardiac disease in ferrets. Semin Avian Exotic Pet Med 1995;4(1):43–8.

76. Edwards JE, Randolph R. Cardiovascular disease in the ferret. Proceedings ACVIM, 1987.

77. Hillyer EV. Ferrets: cardiovascular diseases. In Birchard SJ, Sherding RG, eds. Saunders manual of small animal practice. Philadelphia: WB Saunders, 1994:1335–8.

78. Parrott T, Greiner E, Parrott JD. *Dirofilaria immitis* infection in three ferrets. JAVMA 1984;184:582–3.

79. Supakorndej P, Lewis RE, McCall JW, Dzimianski MT, Holmes RA. Radiographic and angiographic evaluations of ferrets experimentally infected with *Dirofilaria immitis*. Vet Radiol Ultrasound 1995;36(1):23–9.

80. Kemmerer D. The adult ferret. In Proceedings of the Small Mammal Conference. Baltimore: American Ferret Association, 1998.

1. Quesenberry KE, Rosenthal KL. Endocrine diseases. In Ferrets, rabbits and rodents: clinical medicine and surgery. Philadelphia: WB Saunders, 1997:85–98.

2. Fox JG, Marini RP. Diseases of the endocrine system. In Fox JG, ed. Biology and diseases of the ferret, 2nd ed. Baltimore: Williams & Wilkins, 1998:291–305.

3. Rosenthal KL, Peterson ME. Evaluation of plasma androgen and estrogen concentrations in ferrets with hyperadrenocorticism. JAVMA 1996;209:1097–1102.

4. Wagner RA, Dorn DP. Evaluation of serum estradiol concentrations in alopecic ferrets with adrenal gland tumors. JAVMA 1994;205:703–7.

5. Nichols R, Peterson ME, Mullen HS. Adrenal gland. In Birchard SJ, Sherding RG, eds. Saunders manual of small animal practice. Philadelphia: WB Saunders, 1994:238–48.

6. Rosenthal KL, Peterson ME, Quesenberry KE, Lothrop CD. Evaluation of plasma cortisol and corticosterone responses to synthetic adrenocorticotropic hormone administration in ferrets. Am J Vet Res 1993;54(1):29–31.

7. Zorgniotti F. Personal communication, 1998.

8. Aiello S, ed. The Merck veterinary manual, 8th ed. Whitehouse Station, NJ: Merck & Co., 1998:1680–1.

9. Kay ND. Diseases of the prostate gland. In Birchard SJ, Sherding RG, eds. Saunders manual of small animal practice. Philadelphia: WB Saunders, 1994:869–70.

10. Kolmstetter CM, Carpenter JW, Morrisey JK. Diagnosing and treating endocrine diseases in ferrets. Vet Med 1996;91:1104–10.

91. Feldman EC, Nelson RW. Canine and feline endocrinology and reproduction. Philadelphia: WB Saunders, 1987:259, 304–27.

92. Marini RP, Ryden EB, Rosenblad WD, Murphy JC, Fox JG. Functional islet cell tumour in six ferrets. JAVMA 1993;202:430–3.

93. LaBonde J. Gastrointestinal disease in ferrets. Exotic Pet Pract 1996;1(9):1–2.

94. Brown SA. GI disease in the ferret. Proceedings of the Midwest Exotic Pet Seminar, Oakbrook, IL, 1998.

95. Lobprise H. Ferrets—dental management. Proceedings of the Small Mammal Conference. Baltimore: American Ferret Association, 1997.

96. Fox JG. Diseases of the gastrointestinal system. In Fox JG, ed. Biology and diseases of the ferret, 2nd ed. Baltimore: Williams & Wilkins, 1998:273–90.

97. Hillyer EV. Gastrointestinal diseases of ferrets (*Mustela putorius furo*). J Small Exotic Anim Med 1992;2(1):44–5.

98. Williams BH. Epizootic catarrhal enteritis: a novel diarrheal disease in the ferret (*Mustela putorius furo*). Proceedings of the Small Mammal Conference. Baltimore: American Ferret Association, 1997.

99. Dutton MA. Epizootic catarrhal enteritis in ferrets. Exotic Pet Pract 1997;2(5):33–6.

100. Rosenthal K. Gastrointestinal diseases in small mammals. Proceedings of the Annual Convention. Baltimore: American Veterinary Medical Association, 1998:592–3.

101. Bell JA. *Helicobacter mustelae* gastritis, proliferative bowel disease, and eosinophilic gastroenteritis. In Hillyer EV, Quesen-

berry KE, eds. Ferrets, rabbits and rodents: clinical medicine and surgery. Philadelphia: WB Saunders, 1997:37–43.

02. Fox JF, Lee A. The role of *Helicobacter* species in newly recognized gastrointestinal tract diseases in animals. Lab Anim Sci 1997;47:222–55.

03. Li X, Fox JG. Neoplastic diseases. In Fox JG, ed. Biology and diseases of the ferret, 2nd ed. Baltimore: Williams & Wilkins, 1998:405–47.

04. Sleeman JM, Clyde VL, Jones MP, Mason GL. Two cases of pyloric adenocarcinoma in the ferret (*Mustela putorius furo*). Vet Rec 1995;137(11):272–3.

05. Rosenthal K. Interpretation of select clinical pathology values in ferrets and rabbits. Proceedings of the Annual Convention. Baltimore: American Veterinary Medical Association, 1998:602–3.

06. Williams BH, Chimes MJ, Gardiner CH. Biliary coccidiosis in a ferret (*Mustela putorius furo*). Vet Pathol 1996;33:437–9.

07. Blanco MC, Fox JG, Rosenthal K, Hillyer EV, Quesenberry KE, Murphy JC. Megaesophagus in nine ferrets. JAVMA 1994;205:444–7.

08. Hoefer HL. Gastrointestinal diseases. In Hillyer EV, Quesenberry KE, eds. Ferrets, rabbits and rodents: clinical medicine and surgery. Philadelphia: WB Saunders, 1997:26–36.

09. Rice LE, Stahl SJ, McLeod CG Jr. Pyloric adenocarcinoma in a ferret. JAVMA 1992;200:1117–18.

10. Williams BH, Garner MM, Kawasaki TA. Peritoneal mesotheliomas in two ferrets (*Mustela putorius furo*). J Zoo Wildl Med 1994;25:590–4.

111. Blankenship-Paris TL, Chang J, Bagnell CR. Enteric coccidiosis in a ferret. Lab Anim Sci 1993;43:361–3.

112. Bell JA. Parasites of domesticated pet ferrets. Compendium 1994;16:617–20.

113. Rehg JE, Gigliotti F, Stokes DC. Cryptosporidiosis in ferrets. Lab Anim Sci 1988;38(2):155–8.

114. Gomez-Villamandos JC, Carrasco L, Mozos E, Hervas J. Fatal cryptosporidiosis in ferrets (*Mustela putorius furo*): a morphopathologic study. J Zoo Wildl Med 1995;26:539–44.

115. Li X, Pang J, Fox JG. Coinfection with intracellular *Desulfovibrio* species and coccidia in ferrets with proliferative bowel disease. Lab Anim Sci 1996;46:569–71.

116. Fox JG. Bacterial and mycoplasmal diseases. In Fox JG, ed. Biology and diseases of the ferret, 2nd ed. Baltimore: Williams & Wilkins, 1998:321–54.

117. Kreuger KL, Murphy JC, Fox JG. Treatment of proliferative colitis in ferrets. JAVMA 1989;194:1435–6.

118. Miller PE, Pickett JP. Zygomatic salivary gland mucocele in a ferret. JAVMA 1989;194:1437–8.

119. Orcutt C. Dermatologic diseases. In Hillyer EV, Quesenberry KE, eds. Ferrets, rabbits and rodents: clinical medicine and surgery. Philadelphia: WB Saunders, 1997:115–25.

120. Peterson JL, Couto CG. Tumors of the skin and subcutaneous tissues. In Birchard SJ, Sherding RG, eds. Saunders manual of small animal practice. Philadelphia: WB Saunders, 1994:211–15.

121. Parker GA, Picut CA. Histopathologic features and post-surgical sequelae of 57 cutaneous neoplasms in ferrets (*Mustela putorius furo* L.). Vet Pathol 1993;30:499–504.

22. Miller TA, Denman, DL, Lewis GC. Recurrent adenocarcinoma in a ferret. JAVMA 1985;187:839–41.

23. Olsen GH, Turk MA, Foil CS. Disseminated cutaneous squamous cell carcinoma in a ferret. JAVMA 1985;186:702–3.

24. Erdman S. Malignant lymphoma in ferrets. Proc North Am Vet Conf 1993;7:734.

25. Li X, Fox JG, Erdman SE, Aspros DG. Cutaneous lymphoma in a ferret (*Mustela putorius furo*). Vet Pathol 1995;32(1):55–6.

26. Rosenbaum MR, Affolter VK, Usborne AL, Beeber NL. Cutaneous epitheliotropic lymphoma in a ferret. JAVMA 1996;209:1441–4.

27. Messonnier S. Q & A. Exotic Pet Pract 1997:2(4):32.

28. Fox JG. Parasitic diseases. In Fox JG, ed. Biology and diseases of the ferret, 2nd ed. Baltimore: Williams & Wilkins, 1998:375–91.

29. Hillyer EV. Cardiovascular diseases. Part II. In Hillyer EV, Quesenberry KE, eds. Ferrets, rabbits and rodents: clinical medicine and surgery. Philadelphia: WB Saunders, 1997:71–6.

30. Fox JG, Pearson RC, Gorham JR. Viral diseases. In Fox JG, ed. Biology and diseases of the ferret, 2nd ed. Baltimore: Williams & Wilkins, 1998:355–74.

31. Rudling W, Gent N. Aleutian disease in laboratory ferrets. Anim Technol 1994;45(3):149–59.

32. Palley LS, Corning BF, Fox JG, Murphy JC, Gould DH. Parvovirus-associated syndrome (Aleutian disease) in two ferrets. JAVMA 1992;201:100–6.

133. Welchman DB, Oxenham M, Done SH. Aleutian disease in domestic ferrets: diagnostic findings and survey results. Vet Rec 1993;132:479–84.

134. Rosenthal K. Ferret respiratory disease diagnosis. Proc North Am Vet Conf 1995;9:582–3.

135. Rosenthal KL. Respiratory disease. In Hillyer EV, Quesenberry KE, eds. Ferrets, rabbits and rodents: clinical medicine and surgery. Philadelphia: WB Saunders, 1997:77–84.

136. Blair EM, Chambers MA, King HA. Treating distemper in a young ferret. Vet Med 1998;July:655–8.

137. Erdman SE, Reimann KA, Moore FM, Kanki PJ, Yu-Qian Chun Fox JG. Transmission of a chronic lymphoproliferative syndrome in ferrets. Lab Invest 1995;72:539–46.

138. Rosenthal K. Lymphosarcoma in the pet ferret. Vet Cancer Soc Newslett 1997;21(1):10–11.

139. Erdman SE, Moore FM, Rose R, Fox JG. Malignant lymphoma in ferrets: clinical and pathological findings in 19 cases. J Comp Pathol 1992;106:3747.

140. Erdman SE, Brown SA, Kawasaki TA, Moore FM, Li XT, Fox JG. Clinical and pathologic findings in ferrets with lymphoma: 60 cases (1982–1994). JAVMA 1996;208:1285–9.

141. Kawasaki T. Clinical pathology values in ferrets. Seminars in avian and exotic pet medicine. Philadelphia: WB Saunders, 1993.

142. Matus RE. Chemotherapy for lymphoma and leukemia. In Kirk RW, ed. Current veterinary therapy X. Philadelphia: WB Saunders, 1989:485.

143. Hutson A, Kopit M, Walder E. Combination doxorubicin and orthovoltage radiation therapy, single agent doxorubicin and high-dose vincristine for salvage therapy of ferret lymphosarcoma. JAAHA 192;28:365–8.

144. Rosenthal KL. Ferrets. In Quesenberry KE, Hillyer EV, eds. Veterinary Clinics of North America, Exotic Pet Medicine II. Philadelphia: WB Saunders, January 1994:19.

145. Niezgoda M, Briggs DJ, Shaddock J, Dreesen DW, Rupprecht CE. Pathogenesis of experimentally induced rabies in domestic ferrets. Am J Vet Res 1997;58:1327–31.

146. Rupprecht CE, Niezgoda M, Shaddock J, Dreesen D, Briggs D. New frontiers in small mammal medicine: rabies pathobiology in the domestic ferret. Proceedings of the Small Mammal Conference. Baltimore: American Ferret Association, 1997.

147. Lugton IW, Wobeser G, Morris RS, Caley P. Epidemiology of *Mycobacterium bovis* infection in feral ferrets (*Mustela furo*) in New Zealand: II. Routes of infection and excretion. N Z Vet J 1997;45(4):151–7.

148. Schultheiss PC, Dolginow SZ. Granulomatous enteritis caused by *Mycobacterium avium* in a ferret. JAVMA 1994;204:1217–18.

149. Lloyd MH, Wood CM. Synovial sarcoma in a ferret. Vet Rec 1996;139:627–8.

150. Dunn DG, Harris RK, Meis JM, Sweet DE. A histomorphologic and immunohistochemical study of chordoma in twenty ferrets (*M. putorius furo*). Vet Pathol 1991;28:467–73.

151. Williams BH, Eighmy JJ, Berbert MH, Dunn DG. Cervical chordoma in two ferrets (*Mustela putorius furo*). Vet Pathol 1993;30:204–6.

152. Williams BH, Popek EJ, Hart RA, Harris RK. Iniencephaly and other neural tube defects in a litter of ferrets (*Mustela putorius furo*). Vet Pathol 1994;31:260–2.

153. Sleeman JM, Clyde VL, Brenneman KA. Granular cell tumour in the central nervous system of a ferret (*Mustela putorius furo*). Vet Rec 1996;138:65–6.

154. Fox JG. Other systemic diseases. In Fox JG, ed. Biology and diseases of the ferret, 2nd ed. Baltimore: Williams & Wilkins, 1998:307–20.

155. Kirschner SE. Ophthalmologic diseases in small mammals. In Hillyer EV, Quesenberry KE, eds. Ferrets, rabbits and rodents: clinical medicine and surgery. Philadelphia: WB Saunders, 1997:343–5.

156. Miller PE, Marlar AB, Dubielzig RR. Cataracts in a laboratory colony of ferrets. Lab Anim Sci 1993;43:562–8.

157. Gilmour M, Wilkie DA. Diseases of the lens. In Birchard SJ, Sherding RG, eds. Saunders manual of small animal practice. Philadelphia: WB Saunders, 1994:1208–12.

158. Millichamp NJ, Dziezyc J. Disease of the retina, choroid and optic nerve. In Birchard SJ, Sherding RG, eds. Saunders manual of small animal practice. Philadelphia: WB Saunders, 1994:1223–9.

159. Kawasaki T. Retinal atrophy in the ferret. J Small Exotic Anim Med 1992;3:137.

160. Smith W, Stuart-Harris CH. Influenza infection of man from ferret. Lancet 1936;2i:121.

161. Brown SA. Infectious diseases of the ferret. In Birchard SJ, Sherding RG, eds. Saunders manual of small animal practice. Philadelphia: WB Saunders, 1994:1322–6.

62. Fox JG. Mycotic diseases. In Fox JG, ed. Biology and diseases of the ferret, 2nd ed. Baltimore: Williams & Wilkins, 1998:393–403.

63. Bernard S, Leathers C, Bobst D, Gorham J. Estrogen-induced bone marrow depression in ferrets. AJVR 1983;44:657–61.

64. Hillyer EV. Urogenital diseases. In Hillyer EV, Quesenberry KE, eds. Ferrets, rabbits and rodents: clinical medicine and surgery. Philadelphia: WB Saunders, 1997:44–52.

65. Hillyer EV. Ferrets: hematopoietic system. In Birchard SJ, Sherding RG, eds. Saunders manual of small animal practice. Philadelphia: WB Saunders, 1994:1326–8.

66. Mead R, Joseph MM, Neirinckx S. Optimal dose of human chorionic gonadotropin for inducing ovulation in the ferret. Zoo Biol 1988;7:263–7.

67. Gentz EJ, Veatch JK. Cystic ovarian remnant in a ferret. Small Exotic Anim Med 1995;3(2):45–7.

68. Hillyer EV. Ferrets: urogenital system. In Birchard SJ, Sherding RG, eds. Saunders manual of small animal practice. Philadelphia: WB Saunders, 1994:1341–4.

69. Bell JA. Infectious diseases of ferrets. Proc North Am Vet Conf 1993;7:721–2.

70. Fischer PG. Stump pyometra in a female ferret. Exotic Pet Pract 1996;1(10):7.

71. Williams BH. Cystic kidneys in the ferret. Mod Ferret 1997;2(2):31–2.

172. Dutton MA. Treatment of cystine bladder urolith in a ferret
(*Mustela putorius furo*). Exotic Pet Pract 1996;1(8):7.

173. Mann FA, Stockham SL, Freeman MB, Wagner-Mann C,
Besch-Williford CL, Nachreiner RF. Reference intervals for
insulin concentrations and insulin: glucose ratios in the serum
of ferrets. J Small Exotic Anim Med 1992;2(2):79–83.

174. Garibaldi BA, Pecquet Goad ME, Fox JG, Murray R. Serum
thyroxine and triiodothyronine radioimmunoassay values in the
normal ferret. Lab Anim Sci 1988;38:455–8.

Resources

Professional Publications

Atlas of Diagnostic Radiology of Exotic Pets
Small Mammals, Birds, Reptiles, Amphibians
Rubel GA, Isenbugel E, Wolvekamp P
WB Saunders Company
Philadelphia, PA

Biology and Diseases of the Ferret, 2nd edition
Fox JG
Williams & Wilkins
Baltimore, 1998

Clinical Chemistry of Laboratory Animals
Loeb WF, Quimby FW, eds.
Pergamon Press, 1989

Exotic Animal Companion Medicine Handbook for Veterinarians
Johnson-Delaney CA, Harrison LR, eds.
Wingers Publishing
Lake Worth, FL, 1996

Exotic Animal Formulary 1999, new edition
Supplement to AAHA's Practitioner's Guide Series
AAHA, Lakewood, CO

Exotic Animal Formulary
Carpenter JW, Mashima TY, Rupiper DJ
Greystone Publications
Manhattan, KS, 1996

Ferrets, Rabbits and Rodents: Clinical Medicine and Surgery
Hillyer EV, Quesenberry K, eds.
WB Saunders Company
Lake Worth, FL, 1996

Formulary for Laboratory Animals
Hawk CT, Leary SL
American College of Laboratory Animal Medicine

Laboratory Animal Science
Journal of the American Association for Laboratory Animal Science
70 Timber Creek Drive, Suite 5
Cordova, TN

Proceedings of the North American Veterinary Conferences
2614 SW 34th Street, Suite 4
Gainesville, FL
(914) 375-5672

Saunders Manual of Small Animal Practice
Birchard & Sherding
WB Saunders Company
Orlando, FL

Self-Assessment Color Review of Small Mammals
Brown SA, Rosenthal K
Iowa Press, 1997

Seminars in Avian & Exotic Pet Medicine
WB Saunders Company
Orlando, FL

Veterinary Clinics of North America: Small Animal Practice
Exotic Pet I and II
WB Saunders Company
Philadelphia, PA, 1993, 1994

National Ferret Organizations in the United States

American Ferret Association (AFA)
PO Box 255
Crownsville, MD 21032–0255
(888) FERRET-1

Ferret Unity & Registration Organization (FURO)
PO Box 11216
Boulder, CO 80301

League of Independent Ferret Enthusiasts (LIFE)
9330 Old Burke Lake Road
Burke, VA 22015
(703) 503-7313

Legion of Superferrets (LOS)
PO Box 866
Levittown, PA 19058

North American Ferret Association (NAFA)
PO Box 1963
Dale City, VA 22193

S.T.A.R. Ferrets (Shelters That Adopt and Rescue Ferrets)
PO Box 1714
Springfield, VA 22151-0714
STARFerret@aol.com

United Ferret Organization (UFO)
PO Box 606
Assonet, MA 02702

Publications for Pet Owners

The Ferret: An Owner's Guide to a Happy Healthy Pet
Shefferman MR
Howell Book House
New York, 1996

Ferrets USA
Fancy Publications Inc.
2401 Beverly Boulevard
Los Angeles, CA 92718

Modern Ferret
Crunchy Concepts Inc.
PO Box 1007
Smithtown, NY 11787

The Pet Ferret Owner's Manual
Bell JA
Christopher Maggio Studio, Inc. and Miracle Workers
Rochester, NY, 1995

A Practical Guide to Ferret Care
Jeans D
Ferrets, Inc., 1994
PO Box 450099
Miami, FL 33245
(800) 988-0988

Medical Information

Ferret Adrenal Panel
Endocrinology Department
Department of Comparative Medicine
2407 River Drive, Room A105
Veterinary Teaching Hospital
Knoxville, TN 37996
(615) 974-5638

The Ferret Adrenal Panel includes DHEAS, 17-hydroxyprogesterone, androgesterone, testosterone, and estradiol and requires 0.5 ml of serum.[58,82]

Contacts:
Betsy Bailey: bailey.betsy@hospital.vet.utk.edu
Dr. Jack Oliver: joliver@utk.edu

3 French Urinary Catheter available through:[18]
Cook Veterinary Products Inc.
PO Box 2327
Bloomington, IN 47402
(800) 826-2380

Hobby magnifying loupe with interchangeable lenses and cool halo-gen focal light source available from:[57]

MDS Inc.

Brandon, FL

(813) 653-1180

Surgical magnifying loupe available from:[57]

General Scientific Corp.

Ann Arbor, MI

(800) 959-0153

Satinsky neonatal vena cava clamp available from:[57]

Sontec Instruments

(800) 821-7496

Internet Sources

The Ferret Mailing List (FML)

   To subscribe: ferret-request@cunyvm.cuny.edu

Internet Grateful Med: Library of Medicine free search service
   for medical and veterinary articles

NOAH on CompuServe

Pet Care on AOL: advice for owners

Veterinary Information Network (VIN) on America Online

The Veterinary Network: www.vetnet.co.uk

Welcome to NetVet: www.netvet.wustl.edu

Figures

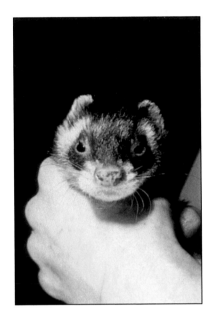

Figure 1

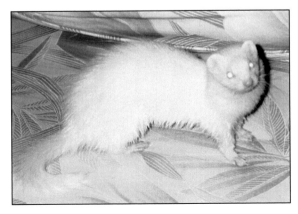

Figure 2

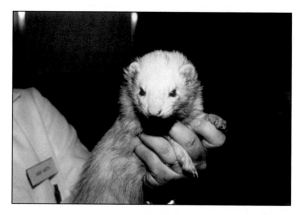

Figure 3

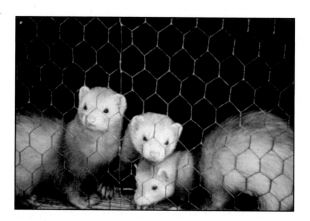

Figure 4

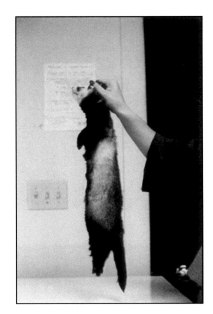

Figure 5

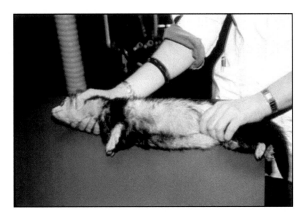

Figure 6

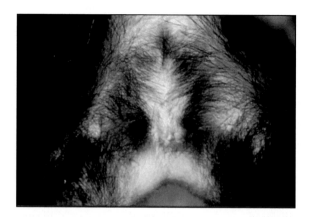

Figure 7a

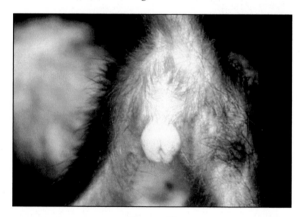

Figure 7b

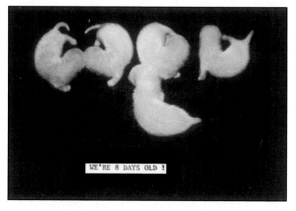

Figure 8

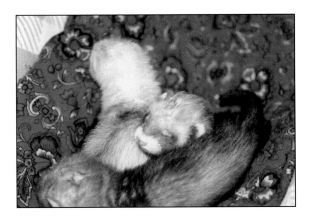

Figure 9

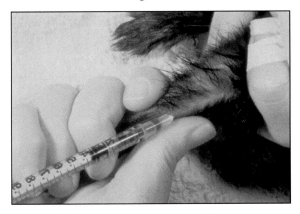

Figure 10

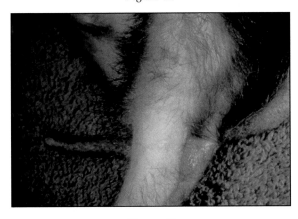

Figure 11

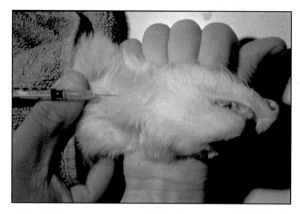

Figure 12

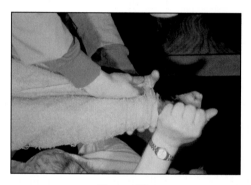

Figure 13a

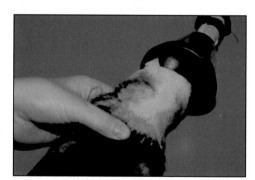

Figure 13b

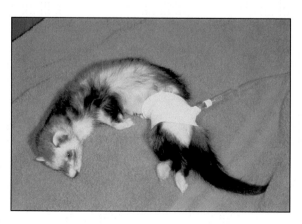

Figure 14

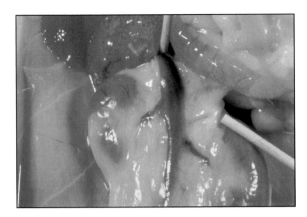

Figure 15

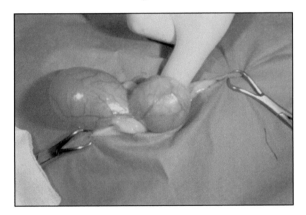

Figure 16

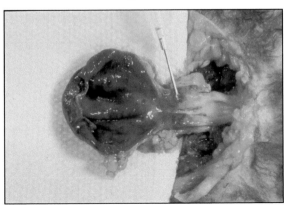

Figure 17

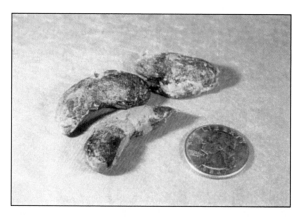

Figure 18

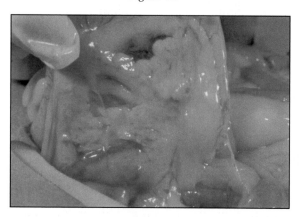

Figure 19

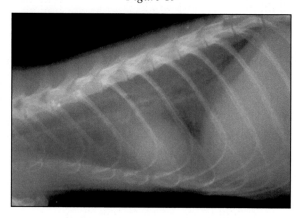

Figure 20

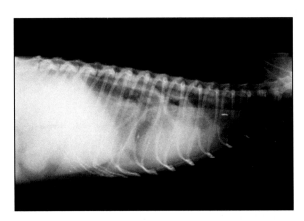

Figure 21

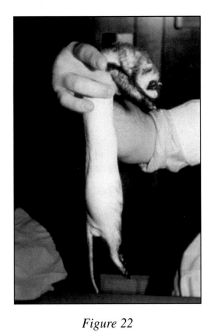

Figure 22

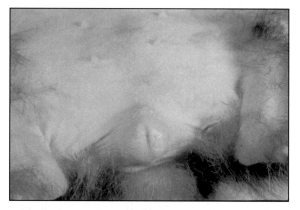

Figure 23

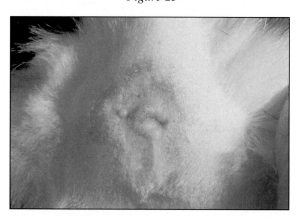

Figure 24

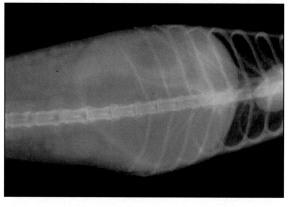

Figure 25

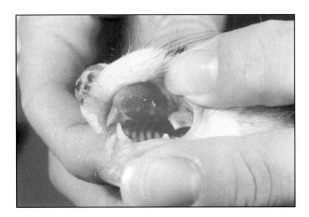

Figure 26

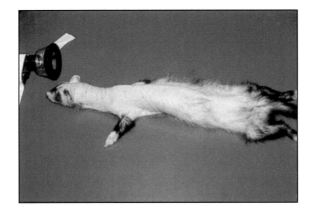

Figure 27

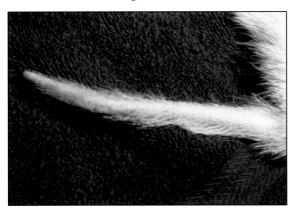

Figure 28

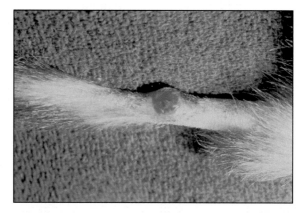

Figure 29

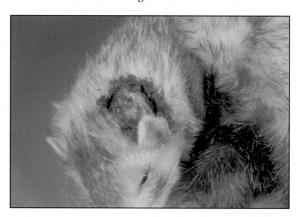

Figure 30

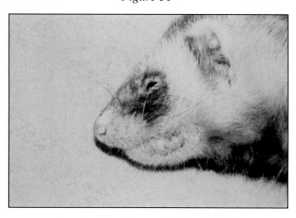

Figure 31

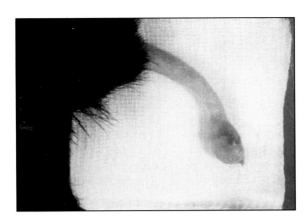

Figure 32

Index

NOTE: Italicized page numbers indicate photos; t. indicates table.

195

Notes